KU-245-054

Acknowledgements

I am indebted to Maggie Goodman, Shelley Gare and all at *Company* magazine who have made this book possible.

I would like to express my sincerest gratitude to Professor Michael Adler, Dr J. M. Emens, Dr Hilary Tillett and Dr E. Wilson-Kay for their kind advice and assistance, and for supplying invaluable information so promptly.

I would also like to thank Lisa Saffron and the Women's Health Information Centre, Peter O'Connell at LBC Radio, Sally Ruth (my friend in New Zealand), Sally Clayton (for typing the manuscript), and Andrea and Carolyn for all their help.

I would also like to express my deepest thanks to all the women who wrote to me and gave me so much encouragement and support. This book is for them.

HEALTHCARE FOR WOMEN SERIES

P. Blanchard.

HEALTHCARE FOR WOMEN

THRUSH
How it's caused and what to do about it

Caroline Clayton

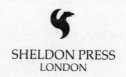

SHELDON PRESS
LONDON

First published in Great Britain in 1984 by
Sheldon Press, SPCK, Marylebone Road, London NW1 4DU

British Library Cataloguing in Publication Data

Clayton, Caroline
    Thrush.—(Healthcare for women)
    1. Vaginitis   2. Candidiasin
    I. Title   II. Series
    618.1'5   RG269.V
    ISBN 0–85969–421–6
    ISBN 0–85969–422–4 Pbk

Typeset by The Bocardo Press

Printed in Great Britain by
Richard Clay (The Chaucer Press) Ltd.
Bungay, Suffolk

Contents

Introduction

Some days I get so depressed. The itching and irritation nearly drives me mad.

When I went to my doctor last month for a prescription I was told I wouldn't have to put up with it all my life – I'd lose it when I got to the menopause. I told him I felt as if I'd had it all my life now. It's not a very comforting thought to think I might have to go on like this for another ten years.

Honestly, it's got to tne stage where I don't feel like a woman anymore.

Second only to cystitis, thrush causes more misery for more women than any other minor illness. Thrush is indeed a most distressing and depressing condition, not least because it tends to recur. Thrush affects us physiologically and psychologically. It changes our attitude to our bodies. It makes us feel ashamed and unclean, and it is a plague on our sexuality. It has probably destroyed the sex lives of hundreds of women and men, and wrecked as many relationships. If you suffer from thrush you'll probably be aware of the great ignorance surrounding it. We need information about the infection and suggestions on how to cope with recurrent attacks. Thrush can be cured – if not with drugs, then with simple, easy-to-use home remedies. And thrush can also be prevented.

This is a self-help book. It explains why we get thrush, how we can get rid of it when we've got it, and how we can avoid getting it again. It also attempts to put thrush into a new perspective – for sufferers and non-sufferers alike. I hope, at least, that it will show anyone concerned about thrush that there is an alternative: there is no reason to suffer anymore.

ONE

What is Thrush?

What exactly is thrush, and where does it come from? Thrush is a fungal infection, rather like athlete's foot, and it is caused by the yeast-like organism, *Candida albicans*. Although the medical name for thrush is *Candida*, it may also be called *Moniliasis*, yeast infection, the whites or fungus. It doesn't come from anywhere. *Candida* is naturally present in the vagina and bowel, along with a multitude of different bacteria and fungi. The acidity of the vagina prevents yeasts and other potentially harmful organisms from multiplying out of all proportion. It is only when the delicate pH balance (acid/alkaline) of the vagina is upset that the 'threatening' bacteria take hold and infections occur.

The warmth and moisture of the vagina provides an ideal environment for the fungus to grow. It is also possible, however, to get thrush in the mouth, intestine or bowel – and in some cases even in the lungs. In fact, it thrives anywhere which is damp and wet. The fungus multiplies rapidly, but, like all yeast, it feeds on and needs sugar to grow, which is why diet plays such an important part in the treatment of thrush. It does not always produce a discharge but is usually very itchy, and makes the whole of the genital area inflamed and sore.

Most cases of thrush arise spontaneously. This really means that they come about because of certain changes which have occurred within the body. Thrush isn't necessarily caught from another person. Babies and little children can suffer with thrush just as much as adult men and women can. However, thrush is sexually transmissible. If you have thrush and you are sexually active, it is very important that your partner or partners are treated too. It is also possible to carry thrush without knowing it since it may not give rise to any symptoms. This is why both partners must be treated for thrush even if only one of you is actually 'suffering'. Thrush may also be transferred by hand, so that it isn't confined to heterosexual relationships.

It is especially important to remember that every attack of thrush, whether it has been acquired sexually or not, can be passed on. More often than not thrush is usually only 'carried' by the male sexual partner. In most, but not all cases, it does not give rise to symptoms. The male here will be a constant source of reinfection unless he, too, is treated. In men, thrush tends to manifest itself as a urinary infection. Doctors call it NSU (Non-specific urethritis). This is an inflammation or infection of the urethra, the tube which carries urine from the bladder to the outside of the body. It makes you want to urinate frequently although there may be little or no water to pass. Urinating is painful, causing a burning or stinging sensation. You may even begin to pass blood. NSU is becoming an increasing concern of doctors in uro-genital medicine. It is regarded as a far more serious complaint than thrush since, if left un-treated, it can develop into Reiter's Disease. This is a form of arthritis which can be crippling. The eyes may also be affected, and some men develop skin and mouth lesions. Like thrush, NSU is frequently recurrent. Women shouldn't ignore NSU because, as carriers, they can reinfect their partner or partners. Men with NSU should always make sure that they are treated for thrush as well, if the attack is linked with it.

This has explained what thrush is. It is important now to make it clear what thrush isn't. First, thrush is not serious, even if it is recurrent. And it does not have complications even if left untreated. In spite of this, however, it is always wise to treat an attack of thrush as quickly as possible since it can prove so difficult to clear up.

Unlike some genital infections, thrush does not make you sterile. It has been suggested that women with thrush may be temporarily infertile when there is a lot of thrush around the neck of the womb, or cervix. If you have been trying unsuccessfully to conceive and have a recurrent thrush problem, it is possible that this may be the reason. Ask your doctor or specialist to check to see if thrush could be a cause.

The fact that thrush is not a serious illness and doesn't have the consequences that, for example, NSU has, if left

4

untreated, helps to explain why some doctors are not too concerned about it. If you suffer from thrush, however, don't ever think that you are wasting your doctor's time. Thrush, particularly when it is recurrent, is a serious problem simply because of the pain and emotional distress it causes. If something is bothering you, go and talk to your doctor and ask for advice.

It can be difficult to talk about thrush. Many women find it hard to talk about their vaginas. Reproductive health care suffers from social taboos and ignorance. Only by talking openly about our problems can we begin to change attitudes. If you are worried about any treatment your doctor prescribes say so. Make a note of all your symptoms and any questions which you want answered. (There is more about this in Chapter 4.)

Secondly, remember that thrush is not *Trichomonas*, another type of vaginal infection. This may seem rather obvious but some doctors confuse the two, especially if they make a diagnosis without an internal examination. Always make sure your doctor has a good look at the symptoms which you describe.

Trichomonas is caused by a microscopically small, one-celled animal. This is the *Trichomonal vaginitis*, and it is only a little larger than a white blood cell. In the human female its normal habitat is the vagina, but it can find its way into the urethra. It does not live in the bowel or the mouth. In men it may be found under the foreskin and in the urethra.

Like thrush, *Trichomonas* may often be present in the vagina with no symptoms. However, when it does cause trouble there is a profuse and intensely irritating discharge, yellowish-green or grey in colour. This has a foul smell. There is more written about *Trichomonas* in Chapter 9, and it is only mentioned here for one reason: never assume that because you have a vaginal discharge that you have got thrush. This holds true even if you have had thrush many times in the past. Only a specialist is able to diagnose thrush with the help of microscopic tests. On the other hand, if you think you have got thrush never let your doctor prescribe you treatment for *Trichomonas* 'just in case'. The importance of seeking specialist treatment cannot, therefore, be stressed enough.

Thrush as an infection, as we have seen, is not serious, but it is a nuisance to all who get it. It is becoming an increasing problem today because it tends to be recurrent. Why it recurs isn't fully understood. Some women, and men, are prone to thrush. Some women may suffer from one, and only one attack in their entire lives. Others are plagued with it. No sooner has one infection been treated and appear to have gone than it returns, seemingly for no reason, with all its previous intensity.

As a sufferer you will get to know what thrush feels like so that you will probably realize when an attack is beginning. For most people the first attack is the worst simply because they do not understand what is wrong. It is very tempting to scratch a furious itch or to soak for several hours in a hot bath and hope that the trouble goes away. Taking this sort of relief is misguided and ineffective as soaking in hot water can actually help *Candida* to multiply, by making the vagina warmer and wetter. Avoid scratching, which irritates and spreads infection.

Here are the sort of warning signals of a vaginal infection: soreness or dryness (it is normal to have a wetness or secretion from the vagina), itching or burning, rashes or sore spots on the genitals, a strong smelling or frothing discharge, a dark-coloured discharge (vaginal moisture is usually clear or slightly milky), an urge to pass water a lot, and pain when doing so. If you notice any of these symptoms get medical help as soon as possible. In the meantime, wear loose cotton clothing. Do not wear nylon underwear, tights or trousers. These may even be the cause of a vaginal infection. Drink plenty of water. Remember that it is possible to abate a urinary infection if it is caught early enough. And most important of all, if you are in any discomfort, abstain from sexual intercourse.

The woman who returns again and again to her doctor with thrush presents a frustrating problem for him or her. Matters are not helped much by the fact that thrush tends to recur almost as soon as the prescribed course of treatment is finished. It may also return after your next period.

Here are some of the most important things to ask yourself about recurrent thrush. They may help you discover why you have got it again. Is the attack connected with sex? Does it coincide with your sexual activity? If the answer to these questions is yes, it is very likely that you are being reinfected by your sexual partner or partners. Always ask your husband or lover to get checked for thrush, and don't start having sex again until you have been given the 'all clear'. Women (or men) prone to thrush could try the sheath as a method of contraception in future to minimize the chances of reinfection.

Thrush can cause NSU. In turn, NSU organisms can cause cervicitis, or an inflammation of the neck of the womb. When one infection begins in the genital area it is very easy for another to follow. Recurrent thrush problems sometimes cease once a cervical erosion has cleared up.

Thrush is mainly a woman's problem, and to understand why women get thrush we need to know a little about the female sexual and reproductive organs. The diagrams on page 8 show these in detail.

The surface sex organs (the vulva) are protected by a pair of outer lips – the labia majora. The urethral and vaginal openings are enclosed within a second pair of lips – the labia minora. The area between these inner lips and the anus is called the perineum.

The close proximity of the anus, vagina and urethra helps to explain why women suffer so much with genital infections. Notice how near the urinary opening is to the vagina. Vaginal infections invariably work their way up to the urethra, and can lead to urinary infections. And once the infection reaches the bladder, it won't be long before the kidneys are affected too. Many infections, including thrush, arise because bacteria from the anus reach the vagina. Hygiene is vital to prevent germs spreading around the vulva. But, as you will see, cleanliness alone cannot protect you against thrush.

The vulva is full of tiny crevices and folds of skin – places where thrush loves to hide. Because of this, treatment concentrated upon the vagina alone is not always sufficient to clear up an attack. Women with thrush should ask for an antifungal cream (see Chapter 5) to smear around the labia to erradicate any fungi that might be lurking here.

So not only does the female anatomy make women more susceptible to thrush, it also makes it harder to get rid of.

External sex organs

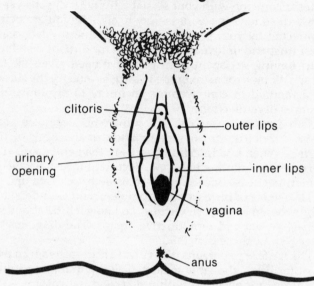

clitoris

outer lips

urinary opening

inner lips

vagina

anus

Internal sexual/reproductive organs

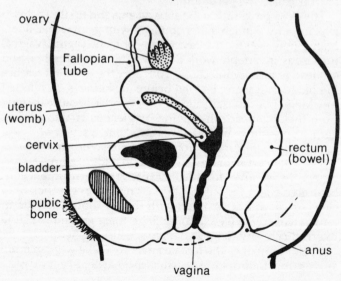

ovary

Fallopian tube

uterus (womb)

cervix

bladder

pubic bone

rectum (bowel)

anus

vagina

What is Thrush?

Men are not so frequently afflicted with it, simply because they don't have a place like the vagina where the fungus can breed so well. When thrush does occur in a man, it will usually have been contracted sexually, and it flares up under the foreskin. This means that circumcized men have even less chance of getting thrush. Remember that it is just as much a man's responsibility to prevent the spread of infection where it can be helped, as it is a woman's.

On a final note, it must be stressed that when you are being treated for any infection, never stop treatment just because the symptoms disappear. It is very important to take a full course of treatment, if you want an effective and lasting cure.

TWO

How Do You Get It?

Imagine for a moment what it must be like, after being perfectly healthy for years, to suddenly develop an illness which you know nothing about. You might never have heard of it before. Not only is this illness very painful, but it refuses to respond to treatment. When it does clear up it seems to return as quickly as it went. Sounds pretty frightening, doesn't it?

For most women recurrent thrush is emotionally devastating. Continual internal examinations are also demoralizing. Thrush makes you feel unclean. You begin to feel abnormal – 'other women don't suffer this way'. You might feel that to be afflicted in this way is some sort of punishment. Life becomes one long course of pessaries. You keep asking yourself 'What have I done to deserve all this? Why have I got it? Why me?'.

The root of the problem lies in the vagina, for this is where the trouble begins. Throughout our menstrual cycle the vagina secretes its slippery fluids. It is normal for the walls of the vagina to feel wet – indeed, it is this moisture which helps to keep the vagina healthy, by keeping it clean and comfortable. The continuous secretion provides lubrication. Without it, sex would not only be less enjoyable, but also uncomfortable.

Vaginal moisture is clear or somewhat milky. It tastes slightly salty and dries to a faint whitish/yellow colour. This may be noticeable on your underwear. The amount of wetness and its consistency varies throughout the menstrual cycle. It increases when we become sexually aroused. After the menopause the vagina loses some of its moisture and elasticity. Usually this only occurs in the latter part of the menopause, about five to ten years after the last period. The lack of fluid can cause irritation so that during intercourse a substitute for the missing lubrication may be necessary.

A dry vagina is far more susceptible to infection. When

the tender mucous membranes are inflamed and sore, infections find it easier to take a hold. This is why it is important not to have intercourse unless you are feeling sexually healthy. If penetration is difficult – and it will be if the vagina is dry or closed up – the delicate tissues are damaged. This makes the perineum sore, and makes a vaginal infection a hundred times worse.

The natural moisture of the vagina has yet another function. It helps maintain the acidity of the vagina and so prevents infections from starting. The mucus secreted by the walls of the vagina contains glycogen. This is a sugary substance. It is fermented into lactic acid by the normal bacteria (lactobacilli) in the vagina. Lactic acid is the same sort of acid as that formed in the making of yoghurt to inhibit fungal growth.

The PH scale

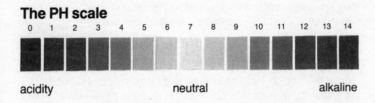

acidity   neutral   alkaline

The natural pH balance of the vagina is usually somewhere around 4.0 to 5.0. During menstruation the pH balance, rises to 5.8 or 6.8 because blood is alkaline. Since thrush and other infections thrive best in the least acidic conditions, you are more vulnerable at this time of the month than at any other.

There are a number of other changes which can take place within our bodies to alter the natural environment of the vagina. Anything that disturbs the flora, or ecological balance, of lactobacilli and other bacteria in the vagina will create conditions which allow thrush and other infections to flare up. And one of the problems in treating thrush with the powerful medicines which the doctor prescribes is that all the good bacteria are destroyed along with the bad. Unless the good ones grow back first the problem will recur.

In summary, the vagina and sex organs are affected by the presence of *alkalinity*, and/or the *lack of protective bacteria*. Fungi multiply rapidly in warm, moist conditions so that *humidity* can disturb the vagina ecology. Too much *sugar* can also cause problems – *Candida* needs sugar for growth. These are the main reasons why we get thrush. If you have a recurrent thrush problem it may be because the infection has never been properly cleared, but is being constantly aggravated by one or more of these conditions. I shall now go on to examine the sort of things that may precipitate an attack of thrush, and which may have a harmful effect upon the vagina.

The pill

Women on the pill are more likely to develop thrush than those using other forms of contraception. There are three types of oral contraceptive: combined oestrogen/progestogen preparations, sequential preparations containing oestrogens and progestogens, and the progestogen-only pill. Oestrogen is one of the female sex hormones. The amount released into the body at any one time depends on what stage a woman is at in her menstrual cycle. It is this amount which helps to make the cycle work. The hormone is present in much higher levels during pregnancy. When you take an oestrogen-based oral contraceptive this has the same effect upon the body as pregnancy. It's quite usual for pregnant women to develop thrush. When you are pregnant there is an increase in the glycogen content of the vaginal mucus. If too much glycogen (sugar) is produced and is not broken down into an acidic form, the vagina loses its natural protection against fungal infections. Pregnant women are thus more vulnerable towards the growth of *Candida albicans*.

Some women find that once the pregnancy ceases, the thrush associated with it seems to vanish. However, this may not be true in every case. And the length of a pregnancy is a very long time to wait to see if the thrush disappears of its own accord. If you are pregnant and are suffering with thrush tell your doctor, or whoever is supervising the pregnancy. Never use an unspecified preparation to relieve your symptoms, however agonising they may be, without asking a doctor's advice first. Don't use up the pessaries you may have at home left over from a previous thrush attack. This is very important because there are certain drugs which should not be taken by pregnant women. Ecostatin, for example, should be used with the utmost caution in the first three months of pregnancy. If you are in doubt about anything always go and talk things over with your doctor.

One of the ways in which the pill works is by increasing the vagina's natural secretions. The thickening of the mucus in the cervical canal prevents sperm from entering the uterus. The additional moisture in and around the vagina can aggravate a recurrent thrush problem. The progestogen-only pill works almost entirely on the principle that progestogen increases cervical mucus. The increased moisture can actually encourage the fungus to thrive! This type of pill has another disadvantage. One of its side effects is heavier and more frequent periods. Break-through bleeding (bleeding between periods) is not uncommon. These may also provoke vaginal thrush. For some women, especially those whose thrush tends to return with a period, prolonged bleeding would be a nightmare.

Cervical eversion

Another of the problems which the pill presents is that it can cause cervical eversion which, in turn, can be a cause of thrush (see Chapter 9). An eversion (sometimes called an 'erosion') means that the soft, red cells from inside the cervix have grown outside. The hormone oestrogen in the pill brings this about. Again, this is a normal occurrence in pregnancy. When an eversion becomes infected – and it will, if you get an attack of thrush – the most effective treatment is to deal with the eversion itself. This can be done in one of two ways: by cauterising, or burning off the layer of cells, or with cryosurgery, or freezing them off. These processes should only be carried out if the eversion becomes troublesome or if infections are recurrent. They are, therefore, valid in the case of recurrent thrush. Both treatments work very well but they don't last forever. Cervical eversion, once it has happened, tends to continue.

There is little use, therefore, in treating an eversion with cautery, or cryosurgery, if the oestrogen which caused it in the first place isn't reduced. This may mean coming off the pill.

The pill is the most effective form of contraception we have to date. For many people it is *the* most effective contraception. Anyone who is considering changing from oral contraception to another sort should of course think the matter over very carefully. For those whose thrush is 'oestrogen orientated', switching to the progestogen-only pill may do the trick in clearing it up. The main drawback in using this particular pill is that it is not so efficient in preventing pregnancy as the other available types of oral contraceptives. There is a much greater risk if you forget to take one of these pills. If this happens the course should be continued as usual, but don't have sex on that particular day. Just to be on the safe side an additional precaution, such as the sheath, should be used until the next period.

I only found out that the contraceptive pill aggravates thrush some six months ago. A specialist suggested that I abstain from taking the pill for a short while. I did so and my condition improved. I went back on a different pill at her suggestion. The thrush infection returned. I stopped the pill altogether at my own discretion. In my case the pill itself was the sole cause of the thrush infection.

I was taking the contraceptive pill for three years before it occurred, having nearly gone mad with itching for three days before I could get an appointment with my GP. TCP cream, I found, eased the irritation slightly, although the aroma wasn't too good.

Anyway, my GP diagnosed my dilemma as thrush – stating that the pill can aggravate the situation. He prescribed a course of six pessaries (Canesten) for three days use. One week later the thrush had returned with a vengeance, so back I went again to my GP, who prescribed a one week course of Nystatin pessaries plus some cream. This luckily worked, but I decided to give up the pill because of the hassle.

If you are thinking about changing your method of contraception it is best to talk about it with your doctor, or

better still, at a family planning clinic. They will discuss all
the options open to you in birth control. The clinic will keep
a constant check on your health through successive visits. If
you do stop taking the pill remember that no other contraceptive will be so easy to use. The sheath and the cap must
be used properly if they are to be effective. This means
using them every time and before sexual contact begins,
whether or not both partners intend to continue making
love until orgasm. The sheath has one big advantage for
thrush sufferers – it is a barrier method. It prevents full
contact between sexual partners during intercourse, but it
also prevents you reinfecting each other. And that can't be
bad!

Sometimes a short break from the pill, perhaps for a few
months, is enough to clear up thrush completely. Even
when you start taking it again, it may not return. It may go
forever.

IUDs

The pill is not the only method of contraception which can
have a disastrous effect on a woman's health. Intra-uterine
devices (IUDs for short) are second only to the pill in preventing pregnancy effectively. They have not been in wide
use for long enough for us to know exactly how harmful
they may be. If the IUD has been incorrectly inserted the
uterus may be perforated. It then becomes possible for the
IUD to slip out of the womb, through a perforation in the
abdominal cavity, where it can cause pelvic inflammatory
disease (PID). If pregnancy occurs while the IUD is in place
it may cause a miscarriage, accompanied by infection.
There is also an increased risk that a fertilized ovum will
become implanted into the Fallopian tube.

Less extreme side effects of the IUD include heavy
periods and bleeding between periods. Allergic skin reactions may occur in IUD users.

Because of the increased risk of vaginal or uterine infections that is associated with the use of intra-uterine
devices, women who are prone to thrush should avoid
them at all costs. The heavy bleeding which may be caused
by this method of contraception, and the bleeding between

periods provoke thrush. If you suffer from thrush and feel that it may be related to your IUD, talk about it with your doctor and try to change to another form of contraceptive as soon as possible. On the other hand, if you use the pill as a method of contraception and your doctor has recommended that you change to the IUD because of thrush, be very wary. Both the pill and the IUD can be responsible for bringing about fungal infections and neither one should really be looked upon as an alternative to the other.

Antibiotics

Many women, and men too, experience an attack of thrush when they are taking, or have just finished, a course of antibiotic tablets. This is because antibiotics cause certain changes inside the body, which make it easier for yeast organisms to take hold.

The term 'antibiotic' means 'life destroying'. It is applied to drugs containing chemicals which are obtained from micro-organisms (moulds, for example). They work by stopping the growth of 'bad' organisms and eventually killing them. They have adverse effects. In destroying any group of bacteria within the body, the balance of micro-organisms in other parts of the body may be disturbed. An overgrowth or superinfection then occurs. This is how anti-biotics cause thrush. And one of the problems with treating thrush, as I have already mentioned, is the fact that in removing the offending bacteria from the system, the good ones are invariably removed too. If the harmful organisms manage to take hold again, the infection continues as before.

If you get thrush when you take antibiotics always ask your doctor, or whoever has prescribed them, if there is an alternative treatment. For some illnesses there may well be. If your doctor is insistent that you take antibiotic drugs, prepare for thrush before it begins. As you take the course of tablets use pessaries or other treatment for thrush as a preventative measure. By taking medication while you are on antibiotics you automatically lessen the chances of an attack getting a hold within the body. In people who are not particularly prone to thrush, such precautions will probably be enough to prevent it developing. But for those of us who seem to spend their entire lives using some sort of treatment for *Candida*, antibiotics spell trouble. This is particularly true for anyone caught in the cystitis/thrush vicious circle.

Cystitis

Cystitis is yet another blight on womankind and female sexuality. Together with thrush it is one of, if not *the*, most common infection to burden women, which is why a book such as this cannot deal with it in full. However, cystitis and thrush go very much hand-in-hand with one another since urinary infections may often be related to fungal ones, and a lot of women who experience cystitis suffer from frequent thrush attacks too, and vice versa. In general, the methods of preventing cystitis are the same as those which tend to keep thrush at bay. These are mentioned later on in this book in Chapters 10 and 11. If you suffer from both cystitis and thrush then it is important to read these parts of the book.

True cystitis occurs when the urethra or bladder becomes infected. Today, many doctors use the term to cover an inflammation of the bladder and all sorts of urinary problems. This ambiguity concerning cystitis is not altogether surprising. When you have a bladder infection you feel as though you want to go to the lavatory every few minutes, although there may be little or no urine to pass. When you do urinate, the urine burns and stings unbearably and there may be blood present (haematuria). Some women whose bladders are inflamed rather than infected – perhaps from vigorous sexual intercourse – experience similar symptoms to these with the exception of haematuria. With each visit to the lavatory, the strain of forcing oneself to urinate has a harmful effect on the urethra. Minute tears occur in its lining so that each trickle of urine along the urethra is agonizing. Whether or not an infection was present originally seems, at this stage, to be of little importance. In any case, with the urethra in a state such as this, an infection is very likely to arise unless the sufferer seeks help.

Escherichia coliform (E. coli) is the germ which causes most bladder infections. It is a natural inhabitant of the bowel, and it causes no problems here. It is only when it finds its way into the urethra that trouble begins. It does not take long for the infection to reach the bladder. From here it may then travel up the ureters – the tubes which carry urine from the kidneys to the bladder. If the infection is allowed to progress this far the kidneys will be affected. A kidney infection is serious, even dangerous. This is why it is important not to ignore the early symptoms of cystitis in the hope that they will vanish of their own accord.

Doctors treat most cases of cystitis with antibiotic drugs. These are very efficient and symptoms usually disappear after a few days. It is important to continue the full course of treatment – just as it is when you are treated for thrush.

Although cystitis may or may not be related to an infection, often it will only clear up with antibiotics. Sometimes, if the trouble is caught in its earliest stages, it is possible to cure it yourself. This involves drinking enormous amounts of liquid, preferably water, usually about half a pint every twenty minutes. However, the intense pain that is associated with cystitis – and all its miseries – is often too much to bear. Antibiotics are then taken when they are not strictly necessary, and the symptoms go away. Antibiotics may appear to be a lifesaver but unfortunately this is not so, as many women have found out. The treatment taken to cure cystitis often results in bringing on an attack of thrush, especially in those who are prone to fungal infections. The fungus, having taken a hold in the vagina, then finds its way into the urethra, and irritates the tissues there which are in the process of healing. The scars in the lining of the urethra open up so that it feels as though the cystitis has returned. Thrush, therefore, can actually bring on another attack of cystitis. In treating the cystitis the thrush will probably return, and so on.

The cystitis/thrush vicious circle can be very nasty and very difficult to break. Even if you suffer from cystitis and as yet haven't been afflicted with the added distress of thrush, the possibilities of this merry-go-round are ever present.

In a way, thrush for me is sex linked. I am prone to urinary tract infections, which I invariably get if I don't pass water immediately after sex. The doctor then treats me with antibiotics, which in turn cause thrush; so the two go hand in hand for me.

I find cystitis and thrush often occur one after the other, the antibiotics for the cystitis causing the thrush to thrive. Most courses of antibiotics have this effect (especially the 'tetra-cyclines'). Also, if I'm run down, the thrush tends to return.

I have suffered from recurrent thrush for several years. Un-fortunately, I have also suffered from a urological complaint requiring surgery three years ago, which has left me with a tendency to cystitis, in particular following intercourse. This requires regular treatment with antibiotics, which in turn leads to another attack of thrush.

If you are suffering from what seems like cystitis, always visit your doctor. Insist that your urine is tested to see whether an infection is present and wait for the results before taking antibiotics – remember, they may not be necessary. In the meantime, try to achieve an effective cure for yourself by drinking plenty of water and urinating frequently so that your system is constantly being flushed through. Mixing a little bicarbonate of soda (an alkalizing agent) into your drinks helps to ease the burning. Stay indoors and try to keep as warm as possible. Placing a hot water bottle against your stomach will help to relieve the pain. This treatment will be more effective if it is begun as the first sensations of an attack are felt.

If you think you can cure your attack of cystitis without a doctor's medicine – this may be relevant for women who suffer from cystitis again and again, who can well recognise the symptoms – try to do so. Alternative treatments to anti-biotics include drinking Mis. Pot. Cit, diluted with plenty of water. Mis. Pot. Cit is an old fashioned remedy for urinary infections. It contains a compound of potassium citrate, and works well, despite its vile taste, because it helps to stop the urine from burning. Mis. Pot. Cit is available over the counter at any good chemist's. Similarly, tablets to relieve cystitis can be bought from health food shops. If you are in any doubt about why you have cystitis or are at all worried, it is always best to ask your doctor's advice. And if your doctor feels it is imperative that your cystitis should be treated with antibiotics, and you are prone to thrush, ask for a course of thrush treatment that you can use at the same time as a preventative measure.

On a final note, remember that where both cystitis and thrush are concerned, self-help will always be the best remedy. And by following the advice set out in this book their tendency to recur can be considerably lessened.

The menopause

Strictly speaking the term 'menopause' means the final period. It is the time when menstruation permanently ceases. For many women, however, this process takes place gradually and is accompanied by a lot of unpleasant symptoms or side effects.

As a woman reaches the menopause her ovaries stop producing a monthly ovum (egg) and cease to produce the female sex hormones, oestrogen and progesterone. The gradual decrease in the supply of these hormones causes changes to occur in the body. The vagina becomes narrower, shorter and hard. The loss of moisture and elasticity in the vagina is called vaginal atrophy, and it happens because of the greatly reduced secretions of the vaginal walls. This in turn can lead to an increased susceptibility to vaginal infection. When the soft inner surfaces of the vagina are damaged – for example, after intercourse without sufficient lubrication – it becomes even more vulnerable. Tears and abrasions provide a place for otherwise harmless organisms to grow out of all proportion.

Hormone replacement therapy with oestrogen can relieve vaginal dryness, possibly preventing vaginitis and other infections, like thrush. Oestrogen creams such as dienoestrol, applied directly to the vagina, may also be beneficial.

Hormonal imbalance

When the balance of the hormones oestrogen and progesterone changes, as it does during the menopause, the secretions of the walls of the vagina and cervix are affected. In fact, in women who have periods, the level of these hormones is continually changing, so that the amount and consistency of a vaginal discharge varies throughout the menstrual cycle. The discharge may increase at ovulation or before a period. The bacteria within the vagina is well adjusted to these patterns and usually no problems occur. The lactobacilli convert glycogen in the vaginal fluid into lactic acid. They maintain the vagina's acidity at just the right level and thus prevent the growth of harmful organisms.

However, if the level of either one or both of these hormones, oestrogen and progesterone, changes dramatically the delicate pH balance of the vagina will be affected. The lactobacilli are unable to function properly and infections can easily flare up. A hormonal imbalance may be contributing to a recurrent thrush problem. Only a thorough medical investigation will either confirm or eliminate this as a possible cause. If you suspect this as the reason why you are suffering, ask your doctor's advice.

Men

Some men seem to have a more alkaline semen than others. This can be enough to trigger off an attack of thrush. Apart from changing your lover, there are other less drastic ways to resolve this problem! A cream like Aci-jel (see Chapter 5) can be used as a lubricant during sexual intercourse. This may counteract the alkaline effect of the semen. Barrier methods of contraception such as the sheath and the cap are obviously a help, especially if they are used in conjunction with spermicidal jellies and foams. These tend to wash out germs and may stop them from growing (see Chapter 6). The pill and the IUD give no protection against infection and may possibly encourage fungal growth.

I was a thrush sufferer for twelve years. My ex-husband also suffered. I now believe that I was not chemically compatible with my husband. During the years that I had it, I would have thrush for two weeks of every four. After the birth of my first child I was completely free of thrush but on resuming intercourse at three months I got it immediately again. I used every pessary on the market, visited doctors, VD clinics etc. Never once was I told not to use tampax or . . . I thought I had it for life, thankfully not. It makes you wonder if I'd stayed with my ex-husband if I'd have ended up with cancer.

I've suffered since 1979, and experienced about six attacks a year. Now I get thrush every two weeks. I must admit it seems sexually transmitted in my case because, if I abstain, I don't get thrush. I did suggest to my doctor that perhaps I was allergic to my husband, but this was poo-poohed! But I got married in 1979, which was when it all started.

Stress

Stress is not an illness. It is a symptom, or rather, a set of symptoms that occur when our body can no longer handle the rough treatment it has been receiving. Many minor complaints, like colds, migraines and backache are simply our body's reaction to stress. If we ignore these danger signals more serious stress-related diseases develop. Thus stress can be the cause of many illnesses – stomach ulcers, diabetes and heart disease, to name but a few.

The causes of stress may be psychological or physical, social or environmental. Marriage, divorce, sexual problems, the death of someone very close to us, and un-employment are psychological stress factors. Minor and/or serious injuries – even pregnancy – are conducive to stress. In fact, anything that puts undue pressure upon us, presents us with emotional difficulties or anxiety, or upsets our everyday routine, can produce stress.

There are times when we all suffer from stress. However, the amount of stress the body can tolerate varies from person to person, so that we don't all react to stress in the same way. For reasons yet unknown, some human beings are better able to cope with pressure than others.

The worst thing about stress is that it can result in illness which then subjects the body to more stress. Thrush is a stress-related disease. Recurrent thrush may be both stress-related and a cause of thrush in its own right. We worry when attacks stubbornly refuse to respond to treat-ment and we thus expose ourselves to more stress. This creates a vicious circle which can be extremely hard to break.

Avoiding stress is the simplest way to prevent thrush if you suspect that these are related. Since there may be two or more factors contributing to a recurrent thrush problem it is usually very difficult to identify stress as a bona fide cause. However, poor health, an inadequate diet, or generally being run down, may provoke an attack of thrush. By making sure that you have enough sleep, improving your diet, and learning to relax, you will increase your stress tolerance level and your resistance to any vaginal infection.

THREE

Some Other Causes

In Chapter 2 I discussed some causes of thrush which might best be called 'medical reasons' – antibiotics, the pill, menopause, cervical eversion, pregnancy and hormonal changes and disorders. If you can attribute your attack of thrush to any of the above reasons then it is quite likely that the problem will disappear once the root cause has been removed. However, if there is no apparent reason why you suffer with thrush, the chances of a rapid cure will be less. Very often it is difficult to identify the cause of a recurrent thrush problem simply because there is a combination of reasons as to why it exists. There may be not one, but many, factors aggravating a fungal infection. If this is so, then almost certainly the cure will take longer and may need a lot of self-help. Establishing the cause of recurrent thrush is usually a matter of trial and error. And sometimes this can only be done by eliminating certain things in your life – one by one – which may be possible causes of the problem. This chapter deals with the sort of things that have become an accepted part of our everyday lives and yet are so detrimental to our health.

Tights and tight trousers

All fungi thrive in warm and moist conditions. Fresh air circulating around the vulva (the outer genitals) is vital. It inhibits abnormal fungal growth. Years ago, when our grandmothers walked around in loose cotton underclothes, thrush was a rarity. The advent of nylon and other man-made fabrics soon changed things. Synthetic fabrics retain moisture since the close weave mesh of their fibres is too fine to allow normal circulating air to pass through it. By wearing nylon pants and tights we are depriving the surface sex organs of the fresh air needed to keep them dry, and to keep thrush and other vaginal infections at bay.

Nylon underwear and tights do not absorb moisture, so

that when the mixture of sweat and the vagina's own natural secretions begins to accumulate, the crotch becomes a very hot and sticky place. In fact, it becomes an ideal breeding ground for thrush and other harmful bacteria.

Tight trousers can also provoke an attack of thrush since they provide a barrier to the air circulation around the genital area, and trap in the sweat from the crotch. Tight jeans also rub together when you walk. The heat generated from this friction can only make the situation worse. Layers of heavy denim are bad enough on their own. When they are worn over nylon tights and pants the effect is potentially disastrous.

Thrush may be caused by tight trousers and/or underwear made from synthetic fabrics. Both make an existing thrush problem much worse and may be the reason why attacks are so difficult to clear up. Don't wear nylon tights, pants or girdles. This is one of the first rules of self-help with thrush. Always wear cotton pants – or better still, none at all where this is possible. Throw your tight trousers away. Wear loose fitting trousers, or if you can't do without jeans, wear skirts on alternate days. And never, never wear nylon pants and nylon tights under tight trousers. This lethal combination is an open invitation to thrush. A thrush attack can build up in a matter of minutes under such conditions.

It is an especially good idea to avoid trousers when you are recovering from an attack, say in the two to three weeks after finishing a course of pessaries. Wearing no pants at all will obviously help here too. A longish skirt will hide all. If you don't feel comfortable like this you could at least forgo your undies in the privacy of your own house.

Soaps and washing powders

Cotton underwear should always be boiled – in plain water. Thrush spores are only killed by boiling, and washing powders also contain harsh chemicals. These can irritate tender areas like the vagina. They can also kill off the valuable natural ecological balance in the genital area and therefore make it easier for the 'bad' bacteria to take hold.

Medicated soaps have a similar effect. They act as an irritant. They are most unnecessary around the vagina since it secretes its own fluids as cleansing agents, keeping it beautifully clean. Washing should help nature – not destroy it. For this reason it is best to cleanse the vagina by pouring cold, pure water over the perineum, but even this isn't advisable more than once a day. If you suspect that your thrush infection is related to *Candida* from the bowel, always wash after passing a stool. Use a little pure soap around the anus and rinse it off with ordinary water. The only other time you actually need to wash the genital area is after intercourse. Pouring cold water over the vulva helps to prevent urinary infections by washing away germs before they can reach the urethral opening.

Baths

While bathing in salt water can be beneficial in treating some vaginal infections, soaking for any length of time in a hot bath can be enough to trigger off an attack of thrush. This is why showers are better for women prone to the infection. Salt baths are recommended for the treatment of non-specific vaginitis when there is very little else that can be done. If you suffer from recurrent thrush, avoid baths. If you must bathe, make it quick and preferably in only a few inches of cool or lukewarm water. Never have a bath during a full scale attack of thrush.

Vaginal deodorants

Vaginal deodorants are an unnecessary hazard, irritating the mucous membranes and possibly provoking an attack of thrush. In any case they cannot work properly since they don't affect germs inside the vagina. Instead, they make it dry and itchy and can cause allergic reactions. Bubble baths and antiseptics should not be used for the same reasons. And perfumed soaps are to be avoided. They kill off the natural bacteria in the vagina in much the same way as antibiotics do.

Some Other Causes

Sanitary protection

Whether or not tampons are a cause of thrush is not fully known. What is clear, however, is that most women are particularly prone to thrush just before, during, or just after a period. Because blood is alkaline it makes the vagina susceptible to *Candida*. If a tampon is left for too long in the vagina, the wad of fibre can become a breeding ground for vaginal infections. And few women could deny that it is easier to forget they have a tampon inside their vaginas than it is to forget that they are using a sanitary towel.

The sorts of fibres most tampons contain are also slightly suspect, particularly those which claim a super-absorbency. Most tampons are made from varying combinations of cotton and rayon, depending on the price of raw materials. Some contain a percentage of carboxymethyl cellulose fibres for extra absorbency. Super-absorbency tampons are rarely necessary except at night, when you keep a tampon in place for a much longer period of time. They tend to have an unnatural drying effect on the vagina, making it more susceptible to thrush and other infections.

Towels may or may not be an alternative sanitary protection for thrush sufferers. If you have recurrent thrush and you use tampons, try sanitary towels to see if the problem improves. Wearing a sanitary towel at night is at least more preferable than using a super-absorbency tampon.

Never, never use tampons or sanitary towels which contain deodorants. And avoid tampons which have plastic applicators. These have sharp pointed teeth which can nick or cut the delicate skin in or around the vagina, and so cause an infection to occur. And be particularly careful if you have an IUD fitted since fibres from a tampon may catch on the string of the IUD. This may give rise to infections.

Natural sponges are an alternative to conventional sanitary protection. Although they are not as convenient to use as towels or tampons they are certainly a lot cheaper. Sponges can be bought quite cheaply from most chemists – in Britain a small one costs about a pound.

It is best to choose one that has tiny holes. Attach a longish thread of cotton to the sponge to make removal easier. Some women find they don't need a string but others do, although the sponge could never be inserted so high that your fingers couldn't reach it. Soak the sponge in water and squeeze it so that it is slightly damp. Once the sponge is in place it should be treated like a normal tampon since it has the same absorbency. When you change the sponge (every two or three hours) don't throw it away. Simply wash it in cool running water, squeeze and then insert into the vagina again. Although there are no problems of disposal you will need to find a lavatory with a wash basin at hand. Buy two sponges so that you always have a spare in case of emergencies.

Sponges are useful in applying acidic solutions to the vagina. They can be soaked in diluted vinegar or lemon juice, yoghurt and herbal preparations and then put into place to ward off thrush attacks. See Chapter 6 on self-help remedies.

Diet

Diabetic women are highly susceptible to thrush. This is because the sugar content in their blood stream is too high. The amount of glycogen secreted by the walls of the vagina increases to such an extent that the bacteria here, whose job it is to convert glycogen into lactic acid, simply cannot cope. Sugar in the urine also gets deposited on the vulva, and so provides fungus with the sweet food it needs to thrive. Where there is sugar, thrush begins to multiply out of all proportion.

Diet plays a vital role in the control of fungal infections. It is important for two reasons: certain foods can actually provoke attacks. We need to know what these are, what way they are harmful and how we can avoid them. On the other hand, by eating other foods we can build up a resistance to fungal infections and actually protect our bodies. Chapter 7 discusses diet in more detail; although it is often only a minor contributor to a thrush problem, it is a complex subject and needs to be carefully understood.

FOUR

Getting Medical Help

The first thing you should do if you suspect that you have thrush, or another genital infection, is to visit a doctor. It is vital to get proper medical help as soon as you can. The longer you allow the fungal growth or bacteria to persist, the more irritating and painful the infection will become. The maddening itch associated with thrush can be embarrassing as well as infuriating – there is nothing worse than trying to scratch yourself in public!

Modern society has left us ashamed of our bodies – not to mention our bodily functions, and there is still a great deal of social stigma attached to venereal disease and to our sex organs in general. When we think we have a genital infection we may be, wrongly, afraid to go to a doctor.

GPs and thrush

Most women who suffer from thrush will go to a doctor for help. In Britain the medical profession is fairly accessible. Everyone living in this country, on a permanent or temporary basis, is entitled to register themselves with a general practitioner (GP). You do not need to pay for an appointment. This service is financed by the National Insurance contributions that we make throughout our lives, in sickness and in health. In other countries, where a National Health Service does not exist, visiting a doctor is not so easy. Nor are the appointments 'free'. When many visits have to be made frequently – as in the case of the recurrent thrush sufferer – this can be quite costly. But the price of ill health pales in comparison with the emotional and psychological trial of repeated visits to a doctor. Arranging one's life around surgery appointments is hardly fun, especially if each visit has little or no result.

You can help to make your visits more pleasant and more fruitful. If you are suffering from an attack of thrush, try to see a doctor at the earliest opportunity. Since it is virtually impossible to predict when an attack will flare up, surgeries operating on a non-appointment basis are better for women prone to thrush. But if you have to wait several days before a doctor can see you, you can ease your discomfort by keeping the vulva as clean and dry as possible. Wear loose cotton clothing. And avoid jeans, tights and baths too. The itching and soreness may be relieved by applying witch hazel to the vulva with swabs of cotton wool. A mild lanolin cream will help to relieve the symptoms until they can be properly treated. Always be wary of proprietary brand creams which claim to stop embarrassing itches. Itching is a symptom of thrush. Don't ignore it!

Many women try to cure thrush with pessaries that they may have left over from previous attacks. Don't be tempted unless you are sure that you have enough to completely clear the infection. Half a course of treatment is worse, in the long run, than no treatment at all. A few pessaries temporarily mask the symptoms and may result in negative swab tests.

Before you arrive at the doctor's be prepared for an internal examination. This is the only way he or she will be able to make an accurate diagnosis. And if your doctor does not want to examine you, ask him or her to do so anyway. It is possible for other conditions to be present in the vagina as well as thrush. The symptoms of thrush can be mistaken for other diseases, and vice versa. Insist on a proper examination before you accept any treatment.

If you are found to have a genital infection your doctor should prescribe some form of treatment, or he or she may refer you to a special clinic or to a gynaecologist. Always ask the doctor what he or she is giving you, how to take it and if it is likely to have any side-effects. If you are unhappy about your treatment say so!

Before your visit make a note of any questions you have about thrush. It is unlikely that you will remember all of the things you want to ask once you are sitting in the surgery. Tell the doctor if you do not understand anything he or she says. And mention anything you feel might help the doctor. The more they know about your thrush problem, the more chance you will both have of overcoming it.

If you suffer from recurrent thrush it would be wise to ask

your doctor if he or she will give you a repeat prescription for pessaries and cream. This will save you and your doctor a lot of time in appointment visits. It also means that as soon as you spot an infection you can start to treat it. You should also use the pessaries at high-risk times – inserting one pessary into the vagina each night during the last few days of your period, for example. If you are particularly susceptible to thrush get your doctor to write 'Not to be given antibiotics, unless essential' on your medical file. This will ensure that you are not advised to take these drugs (when they are not strictly necessary, in the case of a sore throat, for example) on those occasions when you are not seen by your regular doctor.

Always try to make something positive happen from a visit: if pessaries aren't working for you, don't allow yourself to be sent away with yet another course. If you are having little success with your doctor ask him or her to refer you to a specialist. A persistent thrush problem should be thoroughly investigated. Should your doctor admit that he or she can't do anything more for you, get them to refer you to someone who can.

. . . The important thing is that now I know how to cope with subsequent thrush attacks which, unfortunately, I admit are likely to occur. I have confidence in my doctor and her wish to help rather than simply sign a prescription for more pessaries. My advice to other sufferers, especially those people experiencing a first attack, is to go to their doctor promptly. . . As a pharmacy student I would advise others that their local pharmacist will be able to suggest a suitable cream, not to cure thrush but to relieve itching and soothe inflammation before an appointment at the doctor's can be made.

Women doctors may be more helpful since they may have had the same infection themselves. If you are unhappy with the treatment you have been receiving, it may be worth changing your doctor.

Special clinics

If you think that you have thrush you can go to a special clinic (VD Clinic). These offer one of the best facilities for the accurate diagnosis and prompt treatment of all genital infections.

In 1981, a total of 523,319 new patients were seen in special clinics in the United Kingdom. Of these, nearly 51,000 were treated for thrush. Although these special clinics (sometimes called genito-urinary departments) still have some stigma attached to them, only sixteen per cent of their patients actually have a venereal disease like gonorrhoea or syphilis.[1]

In Britain anyone can attend a special clinic without being referred by their own doctor – a situation which does not exist in some other countries. (In the USA, Australia and New Zealand, for example, women with thrush would not normally be accepted for treatment.) Most special clinics now operate on an appointment basis so that it is best to telephone before you arrive. The address of your nearest clinic can be obtained from a family planning clinic, or by telephoning, or asking at your local hospital.

Many people feel nervous about attending a special clinic but the experience should not be a traumatic one. The atmosphere is relaxed and friendly. The staff try hard to put their patients at ease. Complete confidentiality is assured. Remember that the doctors here are experts and they will be able to answer any of the questions you might wish to ask them. You, yourself, must also be prepared to answer all of the doctor's questions with absolute honesty. Your answers will help the clinic to make a correct diagnosis. You will be asked for some basic information about yourself: name, address, age, etc. The clinic will also want to know about any recent sexual contacts, any contraception you are using, and a little about your past medical history.

You will then be examined by a doctor. You will be asked to undress from the waist downwards and lie on a couch, with your legs apart. The doctor will insert a speculum into your vagina. This holds the walls of the vagina open so that he or she can get a clear view of the walls and the cervix. Swabs from the vagina and cervix will be taken. Anal and urethral swabs may also be taken. Cervical smears are

[1] These figures were taken from the *British Medical Journal* 1983: Sexually Transmitted Disease Surveillance 1981, *286*, 1500–1

usually performed as a matter of routine. You will be given a blood test.

It is possible that you will be asked for a urine sample. For this reason, it is sensible to have a full bladder when you attend. Some clinics will ask new patients not to pass water for at least two hours before their appointment.

The vaginal and cervical swabs are examined on a slide and analysed under a microscope so that a diagnosis can be made on the spot. If you have thrush the doctor should be able to tell you so immediately and treatment can begin at once. Sometimes the fungi aren't instantly detectable. Swabs will be sent to the laboratory and you may have to wait up to a week for the results to come through.

The policy of most genito-urinary clinics is only to treat what they find. In effect this means that even if you have all the symptoms of thrush they will not prescribe anything until they have their own microscopic evidence. This attitude may be frustrating for women convinced that they have thrush. It does have its advantages, however. For example, a doctor will often take the patient at their word and will treat that patient for the condition that she or he complains of without carrying out a proper examination. Drugs are powerful chemicals which is why they are so effective, but where there is no infection they can be positively harmful, possibly provoking thrush.

> On many occasions, believing that my thrush had returned, I would go to a special clinic where their routine tests would have confirmed *Candida* if it were present. Because they did not, I had to leave things to calm down a bit on their own. And each time the non-specific infection – which indeed had all the symptoms of thrush – disappeared after a few days. Had I used the strong medication contained in pessaries I would have further disturbed the flora in the vagina, perhaps even bringing on an attack of thrush. In fact, I am sure that the latter happened because of this on many occasions.

Whether or not you are found to be suffering from a genital infection, you will be asked to return for routine follow-up tests. It is essential to attend. It is also important to ask your sexual partner or partners to attend. An asymptomatic male partner may be carrying an infection. Men can harbour thrush spores under the foreskin. Reinfection will occur as soon as sexual contact begins again.

There is a strong link between recurrent NSU and thrush. This is a much more serious disease since, left untreated, it can have severe consequences (see Chapter 1). For this reason alone, sexually active women with thrush should ensure that any male contact is also treated.

The gynaecologist

Recurrent thrush problems should always be fully investigated, preferably by a gynaecologist. Women in Britain must be referred by their doctor. There may be a waiting list for an appointment. If you have to wait several months ask your doctor to continue treating you for thrush until you see the specialist.

Gynaecologists are trained to deal with disorders of women's sexual and reproductive organs. You will be examined internally. You may be asked for a urine sample and given a smear test. As with an ordinary doctor's appointment, it is wise to write down a list of things you wish to discuss with your gynaecologist. Although they can only treat their patients with the same drugs that doctors prescribe, they will investigate a persistent gynaecological problem. They may identify its cause or any underlying factors, previously overlooked by your doctor. For example an irritation on the cervix can be a source of recurrent thrush. A gynaecologist will be able to treat this and in doing so may rid you of thrush.

Well Woman clinics

A Well Woman clinic is a clinic where any woman can go to have a check-up on, and a chat about, her health. They were set up to help women with problems and medical conditions that are often neglected by other parts of the Health Service: cystitis, depression, tiredness, problems connected with periods and the menopause and many others including, of course, thrush. They offer a unique service in health care because the staff (all women) have plenty of time to listen to their patients – with sympathy and understanding. They try to provide information, advice and help so that women can learn more about their bodies and their health. Unlike other clinics that only see patients when they are sick, Well Woman centres will help women who are in good health and who want to stay that way. Great emphasis is put on the prevention and early detection of disease.

Well Woman clinics believe that your emotional health is just as important as a physical problem. They will examine you and give you advice and information about any symptoms that are worrying you. Some of the simple tests that can be done here include those to check your blood pressure, urine, weight, height, and eyesight. And you may be given a cervical smear test, breast and/or vaginal examination. The clinic also provides a counselling service if you have personal problems or family worries that you need to talk about. Well Woman clinics are good news because they offer a more positive support towards mental and social good health.

When you arrive at a Well Woman clinic you will be asked to fill in a questionnaire about yourself and your general health and well-being. This gives the clinic an overall picture of your health and helps them to isolate the areas that are worrying you. You may also be given another questionnaire to fill in and return to the clinic after your visit, to tell them whether the clinic has been helpful and how they can improve it.

You will then see a worker. She will help you to complete the questionnaire. She will have a long talk with you to find out what problems you have and how the clinic might be able to help. She will give you any advice she has and may do some tests. She may want you to see another worker who has a more specialised knowledge – a social worker, marriage guidance counsellor or another type of counsellor. Or she may refer you immediately to the clinic doctor.

Well Woman clinics are excellent places to go if you suffer from recurrent thrush. Although the staff cannot give you a prescription they will examine you to see whether you actually have an infection and refer you to a doctor for treatment. The clinic will advise you on treatments available through your doctor and explain what these entail.

And Well Woman clinics will give you the emotional support that all thrush sufferers so desperately need.

At the end of your visit, the clinic will give you a card. This will be your record of the tests you have had there. If they suggest some simple treatment for you to follow or if the doctor is counselling you for a personal problem, they may suggest you come back to the clinic again to see if your problems are getting better.

At present, Well Woman clinics in the United Kingdom are few and far between. If you want to find out whether there is one in your area, ask at your local hospital; or your District Health Authority or Community Health Council will be able to tell you where the nearest clinic is.

Women's health centres

In countries such as Australia and New Zealand, women's health centres operate on a similar basis to our Well Woman clinics. Many of these have now formed self-help groups to combat vaginal infections like thrush and are helping to remove the ignorance associated with genital diseases in general.

Herbalist medicine

If conventional treatments fail, treatment by a qualified herbal practitioner is always worth considering. Rather than relieving the symptoms of disease with drugs, vaccines or synthetic substances, herbal medicine uses remedies from natural sources to restore good health.

During the initial consultation all aspects of the patient's health are examined. Treatment for recurrent thrush will invariably include a change of diet as well as the use of external poultices with potent anti-fungal agents. Internal medicines to improve pelvic circulation and restore normal tone to the reproductive organs will also be given.

The National Institute of Medical Herbalists is the oldest professional organisation of Herbal Practitioners. A full list of its registered members can be obtained from the National Institute of Medical Herbalists, P.O. Box 3, Winchester, Hants, SO22 GRB, England.

Homeopathy

Homeopathy is a combination of natural healing and medical science. Homeopathic cures encourage the body to fight disease. Treatments are given which would produce the same symptoms in a healthy person as those the patient complains of. By putting more of the disease into the body, the body's natural defences are further stimulated to resist the infection. Obviously, at first, the symptoms of the illness will worsen but homeopathy works on the theory that what causes something can also cure it. Before a diagnosis is made, the homeopathic doctor will examine the patient in depth. Great emphasis is placed on life-style, diet and the condition of the patient's health generally. His or her personality and emotions will also be considered.

Homeopathic medicine is now available, in Great Britain, on the National Health Service. If you think homeopathy may be able to help you, contact the British Homeopathic Association, 27a Devonshire Street, London, W1N 1RJ, enclosing a stamped addressed envelope for a list of homeopathic doctors.

FIVE

Treating Thrush

This chapter outlines the various types of medication used to treat thrush. There are only a certain number available and those who have had thrush several times may well be familiar with all of them. These treatments are the same whether they are prescribed by your doctor or given to you at a health clinic. All of them usually work quickly and effectively. A short course can relieve an attack of thrush within days. Each doctor/clinic will have their own favourite. Similarly, after repeated infections, the thrush sufferer will begin to know which brand works best. If you are prescribed a medicine that you have tried before and have had little success with, don't be afraid to ask for an alternative.

Pessaries and creams

The most effective way to treat thrush is with creams (applied to the infected areas) and pessaries. And in many cases these work well. Cream helps to check the fungal growth, and eventually kill it. Women should use it around the perineum and external labia. Men should apply the cream under the foreskin, on the glans penis and/or wherever it hurts. It offers sufferers fast relief by soothing the inflamed areas and easing the intolerable itching and soreness associated with thrush. Pessaries have to be inserted high into the vagina, preferably at night. These melt fairly rapidly. The potent drugs they contain start to kill off all the fungi with which they come into contact. The number of pessaries needed to clear up a fungal infection varies according to the brand being used. Skin disorders of most kinds are difficult to treat. Using too many potent drugs can lower the skin's natural resistance to infection quite dramatically so that the condition easily flares up again. Most doctors prefer short courses of treatment for thrush victims, lasting from three to six days.

There are several kinds of pessaries which can be used to treat thrush. Of these, Canesten, Daktarin, Gyno-Daktarin, Pevaryl, Gyno-Pevaryl and Ecostatin appear to work best. They are normally used in conjunction with a tube of cream. Containing broad-spectrum anti-fungal drugs, they can relieve thrush symptoms in a few hours, though you are not likely to be completely thrush-free for at least two days. No pessary will offer much protection against recurrent thrush and the last three types on this list have an unpleasant side-effect. The drug upon which they are based – econazole – can sometimes irritate the skin rather than soothe it. As the pessaries melt they begin to sting. This stinging can often be so intense that the sufferer finds it difficult to tell whether it is the thrush or the pessaries that are causing the pain. Econazole, in the form of vaginal pessaries or cream, should never be used during the first three months of pregnancy.

Nystatin (Nystan) is an antibiotic which is active against a wide range of fungi and yeast. In the form of powders, drops, ointments, pessaries and tablets (which are taken by mouth), it is used to treat thrush. Longer courses of Nystan pessaries are needed to cure a thrush attack. These may last anything from one week to one month which is why most sufferers feel unhappy about using them. Keeping to a strict anti-thrush routine for two weeks – no jeans, no tights, no swimming etc – and having to abstain from sexual contact during this time is all very trying. To go a whole month like this, only to see the infection flare up again once the treatment stops is extremely upsetting. Nystan has another disadvantage in that it is an unpleasant yellow colour. The cream and pessaries will stain your underwear. If you have to use Nystan, for any length of time, pantie liners will help to prevent your undies from being ruined.

Vaginal gels

In cases where pessaries of the type mentioned above have failed, some doctors have found that persistent thrush will respond to vaginal gels. These have to be inserted deep into the vagina with a special applicator. Betadine is one such gel. Based on iodine, it is a dark brown/red in colour so that, unfortunately, it will stain your pants. Like Nystan, it has to be taken for long periods of time. This can be a disadvantage but, as most thrush sufferers will agree, any treatment is worth considering while there is still hope of an effective cure.

Oral tablets

Oral tablets may often be given to treat thrush. These work by killing off fungi within the body. Thrush in the bowel or the intestine may be the cause of recurrent attacks. This is particularly true of thrush in the bowel since from here the fungus has easy access to, and can infect, the surface sex organs. As oral tablets work internally rather than externally they usually have little effect in relieving an attack of thrush once it has taken a firm hold in the genital area. For this reason oral tablets such as Nystan should only be taken along with local creams and/or pessaries.

Nizoral is a relatively new type of oral preparation, containing the drug ketoconazole, an anti-fungal antibiotic. When Nizoral was first introduced it seemed as if a major breakthrough in the treatment of thrush had been made. It was, and still is, claimed that Nizoral could clear up *Candida* without the help of pessaries or creams. Trials at the Birmingham and Midland Hospital for Women have found that it is effective in treating cases of acute vaginal thrush and that it seems to work very well.

A course of Nizoral usually lasts for seven days. If you have a bad attack of thrush it is best to take the drug for a longer period of time, i.e. for at least three weeks. And if you are prone to thrush it is useful to continue the treatment during a period, or at high risk times when you are more susceptible to attacks.

One of the main reasons why women find recurrent thrush so difficult to cope with is that pessaries are messy and inconvenient to use. One discharge – the one that is often associated with thrush – is replaced by another, the leakage from the pessaries. And the latter is likely to be more profuse and often brightly coloured as well which can be highly embarrassing and very uncomfortable. In this respect Nizoral and other anti-fungal tablets have a distinct advantage. However, it is worth remembering that they are just about as effective (or ineffective) as are local pessaries in *preventing* recurrent thrush. Once the treatment ceases the chances of another bout returning are as great – or as small, depending on the individual – as they are when pessaries are used.

The adverse effects of Nizoral include nausea, stomach upsets and itching. Nizoral should not be taken during pregnancy.

I've been suffering from bouts of thrush for the last eighteen months, which coincided with my going on the 'pill'. I was given Canesten pessaries and cream. During a four month break from the pill I still suffered several bouts of thrush. After changing to a female doctor I was treated in the same way, but eventually she prescribed an oral anti-fungal Nizoral. This caused the unpleasant side effect of diarrhoea, but since taking a seven day course six weeks ago, I have not suffered any further attacks.

I went along to my GP who prescribed Nystan cream, which controls the itching, and new tablets called Nizoral. The tablets have been out about a year. The course lasts for five days or so – two tablets a day, to be taken with food. This was a tip the dispensing chemist gave me. Otherwise, she said, they don't work, because the acid secreted during digestion is necessary for them to be effective.

Medicated powders

Thrush is also treated with medicated powders, such as Nystan or Mycil. In general, powder is more beneficial for men. Its drying effect helps to relieve the inflamed skin. Women can use powder around the vulva, although it should not be applied inside the vagina. Anti-fungal powders are quite pleasant to use. A frequent dusting down in the genital area would seem an ideal way of helping to prevent recurrent bouts of thrush. By regularly using an anti-fungal powder men can play a positive role in helping to rid women of recurrent thrush problems.

Medicated tampons

Medicated tampons are another alternative to pessaries and vaginal gels. In fact, they appear to have a high success rate, which is very encouraging news for all victims of thrush. In addition to this they have other advantages over the treatments which have so far been discussed. They are pushed high into the vagina exactly like normal tampons. Inserted either at night or during the day, they remain in close contact with the source of the thrush for a relatively long period of time, longer than other medications such as pessaries do. Medicated tampons can be used during a period instead of ordinary tampons. They are, therefore, ideal for women whose thrush tends to recur after a period, or for sufferers who become more susceptible towards fungal infections during menstruation. Vaginal pessaries and gels tend to be messy, whereas tampons keep the medication inside the body. Many doctors seem reluctant to prescribe medicated tampons despite their high success rate. This could be because they are relatively expensive when compared with other forms of treatment. Or perhaps simply because their relative merits have not yet been recognised. Whatever the reason it is worth trying medicated tampons, just as it is worth getting to know all the available treatments. If you have a persistent thrush problem which has so far shown little response to various sorts of pessaries or gels, this type of medication may be your answer.

> Although I still suffer at least three or four times a year now I have found a cure. They are called Gyno-Daktarin tampons and were prescribed by a visiting lady doctor at my local surgery. They are tampons which contain the ingredients of pessaries, are less messy, and they work for me.

Gentian violet

Painting the vagina and cervix with gentian violet is an old-fashioned remedy still used by doctors to treat women prone to vaginal infections like thrush. It is often very effective. It is also very simple, painless and cheap. Available over the counter at any good chemist's, gentian violet can be used at home as a preventative measure against thrush. (It is important to ask for an aqueous solution, and not alcohol which will burn.) It can be inserted into the vagina with a contraceptive foam applicator or on a tampon. Doing this once a day for two or three days is sometimes enough to abate a mild attack. However, be warned – it is very messy! Gentian violet contains a purple dye that will stain anything with which it comes into contact. For this reason it is best to use it in the bath or shower. Should any of the liquid splash onto the enamel, wash it off at once. Avoid getting it on towels, flannels, and also your hands. And wear a tampon or sanitary towel for the next few days to protect your underwear.

Lactic acid

Lactic acid pessaries – Lactinex – used to be available from chemists. Sadly, since they are no longer as popular as they were, they have become more difficult to obtain. This is a great pity. Although lactic acid is one of the oldest treatments for thrush it is no less effective than the most modern ones. It works by restoring the natural acidity of the vagina – remember that thrush and other fungi cannot grow in an acidic environment. Lactic acid is, however, still available in its liquid form and sufferers can use it as part of their self-help routines. Using it with a little lactic acid diluted with water may help to prevent an attack of thrush. Alternatively, you could have a very brief soak in a bath containing diluted lactic acid.

Aci-jel

Aci-jel is called a 'therapeutic vaginal jelly'. Like lactic acid, it can be bought at the chemist's and it works in exactly the same way – by making the vagina less favourable to thrush. Again, it is best used as a preventative measure against thrush.

I have suffered from thrush, on and off, for over a year now. The first time I saw a doctor he prescribed a bottle of Nystatin pills and some Nystatin cream. The cream was useless and the pills

43

were only effective while I was taking them. The second time I went I saw a female doctor . . . She explained the cause and, after a long discussion, she prescribed a therapeutic vaginal gel. This treatment is a bit more successful, although the method of application sometimes puts me off using it.

Cryosurgery

Cryosurgery can also be regarded as a 'cure' for thrush. As I have mentioned in Chapter 3, many thrush problems are related to cervical irritation. Once an eversion has become troublesome it becomes more difficult to clear up thrush and other infections present in the vagina. Treating an eversion with cautery or cryosurgery will reduce the likelihood of further attacks of thrush.

Problems with prescribed treatments

Although thrush has a strong tendency to return, for some people the first attack may well be the last. This is usually true where the infection has arisen from a direct cause, such as a course of antibiotics. But for many others, thrush can recur again and again, lasting for several months at a time. Men and women who are less fortunate have found themselves burdened with a recurrent thrush problem for years.

It is important to remember that none of the treatments mentioned here offers a permanent cure for thrush. While they are nearly all capable of clearing up an attack once it has taken hold, only self-help will prevent further infections developing.

The problem with treating thrush with powerful chemicals is that the medication removes all of the good bacteria present in the vagina along with the bad. Unless the good ones grow back first the bad will trigger off another infection. Destroying the sex organs' delicate flora, or ecological balance, only makes them more vulnerable to infection. This is why self-help is so important.

SIX

Self-help Remedies

Self-help remedies are an alternative to a doctor's powerful drugs. There are a number of ingredients that can be used at home to cure and prevent attacks of thrush, and most of these can be found in the food cupboard. Vinegar, yoghurt and many different types of herbs have been used by women for centuries to combat vaginal infections. Unlike the medication that doctors prescribe which tends to destroy all bacteria – the good along with the bad – self-help treatments work by restoring the vaginal ecology. Self-help with thrush allows you to help your body to heal itself.

Home remedies may be particularly valuable to the sufferer of *recurrent* thrush and other vaginal infections. Where conventional medicines have failed, it may be that natural therapy will succeed. Obviously not all of the solutions described here will work for everyone. What will work for one woman at one time may be ineffective for that same woman on another occasion. However, self-help remedies are easy to use, cheap and have little or no side effects. While they may not do any good, they cannot, on the other hand, make the problem any worse. And all of them are worth giving a try.

Most of the remedies described here are liquid solutions. Introducing them into the vagina, and getting them to stay there, presents a tricky problem. Here are some methods that you could try:

- Put the solution into the vagina using a spermicide applicator, or in a cap or diaphragm.

- Dampen cotton wool balls in the solution and insert them into the vagina in a diaphragm.

- Dip or soak a tampon in the mixture/solution, insert into the vagina and leave in place overnight.

- Place a soaked tampon in a diaphragm, fold it together, and insert it as usual.

45

Some of the remedies mentioned in this chapter can be poured into a few inches of bath water. Sit in the bath with your knees apart. Open your vagina by gently inserting a finger or two, pulling down slightly to allow the water to run in.

Yoghurt

Yoghurt is one of the oldest known and most effective treatments for yeast infections like thrush. It works because it contains cultures of *lactobacilli*, a type of bacteria naturally present throughout the body. In the vagina it plays an important part in keeping *Candida* and other organisms under control. Lactobacilli breaks down the glycogen content in the vaginal secretions, converting it into lactic acid. This process keeps the vagina fairly acidic so that potentially harmful bacteria like thrush, which thrive best in alkalinic environments, die. Vaginal infections occur when this delicate acid/alkaline balance is disturbed. Thrush, for instance, indicates that the vagina is too alkaline. Lactobacilli cultures can restore the natural acidity of the vagina and so promote healing.

Plain unpasteurised yoghurt is the best source of lactobacilli. Only natural yoghurt, with a live acidophilus culture, and not the flavoured, fruity variety, will be effective.

To combat fungal infection yoghurt should both be eaten and applied directly to the vagina and perineum (or used in a solution). Attacking the problem from both ends lessens the likelihood of reinfection since the fungus which causes thrush can develop and grow in the intestine. An attack of vaginal thrush may indicate that the fungus is present in the intestine too. This can be corrected within a few days by eating lots of yoghurt or acidophilus milk or culture.

In all cases yoghurt should be used at the first signs of infection. Use natural yoghurt (live) directly, inserting it into the vagina twice a day for about a week. Rubbing plain yoghurt on the irritated skin around the vagina will help to soothe the inflammation.

To make a yoghurt solution add about two or three tablespoons of plain yoghurt to two pints of warm water. Use daily for up to a week. Alternatively, buy acidophilus culture from a health food store. This contains a lactobacilli culture in liquid form. Use this twice a day for one week. Acidophilus capsules can be bought from health food shops. Insert one into the vagina twice a day for one week.

Many women find that by using yoghurt at the first signs of infection, an attack of thrush can be relieved within hours. Usually it will disappear after only a few days of treatment. If, however, the symptoms still persist after a week, it is best to stop treating it yourself and to visit a doctor.

After having thrush on and off for two years I solved my problem by changing from the pill to the cap, and using yoghurt to treat the residual infection, having had no joy with Nystan pessaries. This I applied either in my cap or with tampons for about ten days. (I used, of course, natural yoghurt.) I've finally got rid of thrush.

I too was a sufferer – intermittently for about four years, significantly, while I was on the pill. I was treated with antibiotic pessaries when I eventually plucked up courage to seek treatment, but wasn't happy about it. A young female GP suggested an old-fashioned remedy – *natural yoghurt*! Instant success and relief within a few hours – if a trifle messy!

Vinegar

Vinegar, and to an extent lemon juice, help to restore the acid balance of the vagina. Using weak solutions of vinegar and lemon juice can sometimes cure an attack of thrush. Vinegar and salt solutions are also helpful in treating non-specific vaginal infections.

Use about two tablespoons of white, sugarless vinegar or lemon juice to one pint of water. Soak a tampon in this solution and then insert into the vagina overnight. You could try pouring a little vinegar into a few inches of bath water and sitting down in it for about five minutes, but remember that long soaks in hot water can do more harm than good.

Salt is a neutralizing agent. Salt baths are therapeutic as they help to soothe and heal inflamed mucous membranes.

For a non-specific infection, alternate vinegar and salt water solutions for a week. Use the vinegar solution one day, the salt water solution the next and so on. Add about half a tablespoon of salt (or two tablespoons of vinegar) to every pint of water that you use.

Bicarbonate of soda

Some women have found relief from thrush with bicarbonate of soda, either in the form of sodamints (indigestion tablets) inserted high into the vagina, or simply by diluting the bicarbonate in their bath water. Treating thrush in this way is slightly unusual. Other cures work by making the vagina more acidic – too acidic for *Candida* to grow in. Bicarbonate of soda is used to increase the vagina's alkalinity so that it is too alkaline even for the fungi to survive.

Sodamints are difficult to obtain since they have gone out of fashion in recent years. Some chemists may still stock them, however, and certain pharmacists may be prepared to make them up for you. Certain health food stores may also be able to help. Otherwise, add a little bicarbonate of soda to the bath water, or use with a mild solution of bicarbonate of soda and cool water.

Garlic

Garlic is well known for its healing properties. It is a form of antibiotic. It has been used for centuries by women to treat vaginal infections.

Garlic may, or may not be, a specific cure for thrush but it will help non-specific vaginitis, and may also be useful when more than one infection is present in the vagina at any one time.

- Put eight cloves of garlic in a jar with about half a pint of white, sugarless vinegar. Leave this by a window for about two days, until the oil of the garlic has been released. Use a tablespoon of this solution in one pint of water. Use twice a day for a week.

- If an irritation develops then just use a garlic solution; boil a pint of water and add a peeled and chopped garlic clove. Boil together for about fifteen minutes, strain and leave to cool. Use twice a day for a week.

- Garlic cloves can be inserted into the vagina, and perhaps in this way, work more effectively. Slice a clove in half. Wrap it in gauze. Insert into the vagina and leave overnight.

Spermicides

Spermicidal jellies and foams are a useful form of contraceptive when they are used correctly in conjunction with the sheath or cap. They *may* protect women against some sexually transmitted diseases like gonorrhoea, and *may* offer protection against cancer of the cervix. They *may* also help to prevent vaginal infections like thrush. It's possible that they inhibit bacterial and fungal growth. They can be bought from any chemist and used as a preventative measure against thrush. Some women, however, develop an allergic reaction to spermicides (see Chapter 9), and they can actually be the source of a vaginal infection.

Herbs

Here are some simple herbal remedies that are effective in curing and preventing thrush. Like most self-help remedies they work by restoring the body to its normal environment, and again, are inexpensive. Herbal solutions can be inserted into the vagina. It is also possible to make poultices (herb-soaked pads) which help to relieve the external itching and soreness associated with thrush, while they fight the infection inside.

You can use fresh or dried herbs. Buying in bulk is cheaper. To prepare a herbal solution, boil the specified amount of herb (usually a half to one ounce) in about two pints of water. Strain the liquid and always allow it to cool before use. Never use aluminium utensils to prepare herbs.

Herbal Solutions

1. Bayberry Bark: Boil two pints of water. Add two to three tablespoons of bayberry bark, and boil gently for about twenty minutes. Strain the liquid and leave to cool. Use daily for a week.

2. Goldenseal and Myrrh: Boil one and a half pints of water. Add a tablespoon of goldenseal and one tablespoon of myrrh. Simmer for twenty minutes. Strain the liquid. Use daily for a week to treat thrush and/or *Trichomonas* (see Chapter 9).

   Goldenseal is also good for any vaginitis. Boil a pint of water. Add one teaspoon of goldenseal powder. Simmer for twenty to thirty minutes. Add enough water to make up two pints in total. Use daily for one week.

3. Thuja: Thuja is an anti-fungal herb. It is available as an ointment from health food shops and herbalists. This can be smeared on to a tampon or added to water to make a solution. Ten drops of thuja diluted in a glass of water can also be drunk three times daily.

   Calendula (marigold), slippery elm, black willow bark, pit root and fennel seed, rosemary and sage can be used to treat all non-specific vaginitis. Chickweed, chapparral and chamomile are effective in treating *Trichomonas*.

Herbal Poultices

Herb soaked pads can be held to the genital area for five minutes to several hours to relieve external itching. To make a herbal poultice use fresh herbs wrapped in muslin or cotton. Dampen the pad slightly, and change when it becomes dry.

Cottage Cheese

Cottage cheese wrapped in muslin, and worn on a sanitary towel daily for two weeks can be helpful in treating thrush. The cheese relieves the itching and soreness associated with thrush and apparently helps to draw the infection out of the system. This poultice should be changed several times a day, according to the severity of the attack. It is reported to be most effective when oatstraw tea is drunk daily.

Oatstraw Tea
Add one teaspoon to one cup of boiling water. Drink daily for a month while you are being treated for a fungal infection. A stronger tea, allowed to steep for fifteen minutes, can be used as a poultice or added to the bathwater.

Some other points

Drinking cranberry juice and/or one teaspoon of vinegar and one teaspoon of honey in hot water helps by creating a more acidic environment within the body.

Herbal remedies are potent. If one is going to work it will have done so within a week. It is best to use these treatments at the first signs of an infection and to continue to do so for the next seven days. If after this time you still think you have an infection, see a doctor.

Although thrush is not a serious disease it is important to treat it at its first signs. The symptoms of thrush are such that they can easily be confused with other infections. Vaginal discharge, irritation and soreness could indicate a multitude of infections from non-specific vaginitis through to more serious diseases like gonorrhoea. Similarly two or more infections may also be present in the vagina alongside of thrush. They need to be properly diagnosed and appropriately treated. It is, therefore, imperative to visit a doctor before you attempt to treat an infection yourself, however mild or acute the symptoms may be.

SEVEN

Diet

> I have been plagued with thrush for the last six months but was
> not aware then what it was. I did not approach a doctor until the
> itching made me totally miserable. I was treated with a vaginal
> cream but it never actually cleared up. I was still having a
> discharge and itching and was particularly worse on days after
> I'd eaten nothing but sweet things and not a proper meal.

Of all the information about self-help measures which we
can take to protect ourselves against thrush, dietary advice
seems to be the hardest to obtain. Diet plays a vital role in
helping to safeguard the body against illness. And yet how
many of us have ever been warned that the foods we eat –
or aren't eating, as the case may be – are contributing to a
recurrent thrush problem?

A sensible diet should keep us in good health. An attack
of thrush is often a sign of poor eating habits. By re-
assessing the value of the things we eat, we can take a
positive step forward in helping ourselves to better health.

What is a healthy diet? Food is needed for energy and for
the growth and maintenance of the human body. Protein,
fat, and carbohydrate are the three basic nutrients which
can provide this energy. All foods contain various amounts
of proteins, fats and/or carbohydrates. Some foods are high
in vitamins and minerals that are essential for good health.
They help to prevent disease and keep our blood and tissue
fluid functioning. They keep our skin and our hair in good
condition, and much more besides.

A healthy diet must be a balanced diet. It should contain
all of the nutrients our body needs – proteins, fats, carbohydrates, vitamins and minerals. A diet which lacks one or
more of these requirements may have quite serious short-
term or long-term effects. For example, carbohydrates are
very important because they assist in the assimilation and
digestion of other foods. Fat and carbohydrate (sugar) are
both sources of energy, but fat cannot easily be burnt off

without the presence of sugar. Protein is primarily a body 'builder'. It is utilised by the body to repair and build up the skin, the hair, the muscles and all of our internal organs too. When we eat less fat and carbohydrate, protein has to be used to provide energy, though it may be badly needed for repairing and replacing damaged cells within the body.

People in the western world today eat a large proportion of refined or processed foods. These have little of the nutritional content of fresh, untreated foods. Valuable vitamins and minerals are lost during the refining process. And convenience foods lack the roughage or fibre which the body needs to get rid of its waste products.

Refined sugar has become an accepted part of our lives. We eat too much of it. We take it in our tea and coffee, in soft drinks like cola and lemonade, and in cakes, sweets and chocolate bars. We have developed a 'sweet tooth' and consequently our health suffers.

An excessive amount of sugar in the diet can be dangerous for several reasons: it interferes with the absorption of proteins, calcium and many other minerals, it destroys the valuable bacteria that live in our intestines which help to keep us healthy, too much sugar over-stimulates the production of insulin and can cause diabetes, and sugar is the great aggravator of thrush.

The sugar/thrush connection

The mucous membranes of the vaginal walls secrete glycogen, a sugar compound. Bacteria which live in the vagina, called lactobacilli, ferment this sugar into lactic acid. This process inhibits fungal growth and keeps vaginal infections at bay. It maintains the pH balance of the vagina at just the right level, so that it is too acidic for thrush and other organisms to survive in.

The intestines are populated by the same sort of bacilli. They are invaluable here. They, too, feed on sugar and produce lactic acid to destroy potentially harmful organisms fighting for survival in the gut. Similar bacteria are present in the mouth, working to the same ends. They break down sugar, forming lactic acid in the process. It is this acid which causes tooth decay – another reason for avoiding sugar and sweets!

Eating large quantities of sugar has a negative effect on our intestinal, vaginal and oral bacteria. Lactobacilli are unable to cope with the amount of sugar in the intestinal tract. They cannot ferment all the sugar into lactic acid. They cannot suppress the disease – and odour-producing-bacteria which surround them. Once the 'bad' organisms gain a hold in the body, they multiply out of all proportion, using the sugar to their advantage – fungi thrive on sugar.

An abundance of thrush in the gut and bowel will soon infect the vagina. A general absence of 'good' bacteria throughout the body stimulates the growth of thrush anywhere – in the mouth, in the stomach, in the bowel and in the vagina. This is the sugar/thrush connection. Sugar not only destroys beneficial organisms in the body; it also encourages degenerative bacteria to grow. Recurring thrush may be caused by a high carbohydrate intake.

Carbohydrates

There are many sources of sugar in the diet. All of these sources are classed as carbohydrates; a group of foods which contain sugar, starch and/or cellulose. During digestion all starch is converted into sugar, and all sugar is then broken down into glucose. In this form, starches and sugars can be absorbed into the bloodstream. Some glucose is used in the tissues to provide energy wherever it is required. The remainder is recombined to form glycogen. This can be stored in the liver and muscles until it is needed. As the level of glucose in the blood begins to fall, glycogen stores are released and broken down again. The level of glucose in the bloodstream is carefully regulated by this process.

Although all carbohydrate foods are eventually converted into sugar there are certain foods in this group which are 'better' than others. These are called superior carbohydrates. They are supplied by root vegetables, wholegrain breads and cereals, and fresh fruits. They are 'better' because in these foods the conversion of starch into sugar is gradual. Sugar is released slowly, in quantities that the intestinal bacteria can manage. Superior carbohydrates are particularly high in vitamins and minerals, and in cellulose. Cellulose has little energy value but provides fibre to help the body eliminate its waste products. These foods, in modest amounts, are valuable and necessary in our diet. And there is no reason why they should be avoided.

If you suffer from recurrent thrush you should cut down your intake of refined foods. These tend to be the worst carbohydrate source. They contain little or no fibre. The amount of vitamins and minerals they supply is greatly reduced during the refining process. Many women find that an attack of thrush occurs after they have been over-indulging in sweets, cakes and biscuits.

Without eating refined sugar in any form, a combination of natural sugars and sugar-formers together with the sugar freed during the digestion of starch brings our total sugar intake up to a surprisingly large amount. When we eat foods of a high carbohydrate content we can consume more than a pound of sugar a day. And this doesn't even take into account the sugar we might heap into our hot drinks, or on to our morning cereal as well! Other foodstuffs are deceptively high in sugar: baked beans, bananas, figs, macaroni, noodles, plums and prunes, and particularly canned and dried fruits.

By eating sensibly we can help our bodies to fight infection and we can prevent recurrences of vaginal thrush. Always be wary of refined sugars, flours, cereals and breads. In effect, this means avoiding most of the things we love to eat – chocolate, cakes, sweet sauces, jams and marmalades. White bread, rolls and buns, and white flour, packaged cereals, rice and pasta should be replaced with brown, whole-grain foods.

To keep thrush at bay, and to keep healthy, choose your carbohydrate intake from those foods which have an unusually low sugar content: asparagus, beets, brussels sprouts, cabbage, carrots, cauliflower, celery, cucumbers, kale, leeks, lettuce, dried onions, green peppers, pumpkin, radishes, rhubarb, spinach, string beans, tomatoes and watercress. These foods are also low in calories and contain lots of vitamins and minerals.

Diabetes

Diabetic women are highly susceptible to thrush owing to the high or uncontrolled levels of sugar in their blood. Diabetes means that the body is unable to break down and use its foods properly. This is because diabetics are either deficient in insulin – a hormone secreted by the pancreas – or because their bodies do not react properly to the insulin they produce. Insulin makes it possible for sugar (glucose) to enter the cells to be converted into energy. Since this sugar can neither enter the cells nor be utilized as energy, it accumulates in the bloodstream. When the glucose level gets too high, sugar spills into the urine. The kidneys have to provide more urine to carry this glucose. The body needs to replace the excessive amounts of urine that the diabetic produces. Severe thirst and an increased need to urinate are the earliest symptoms of the disease.

Women with diabetes have extra sugar in their vaginal walls which encourages the growth of thrush. Sugar in the urine, deposited on the vulva, provides food for the fungus. Undetected diabetes may be the source of a recurrent thrush problem. And unless the diabetes is brought under control it is very likely that the thrush will continue to be a problem.

Diabetes can be treated. Some patients will need a large daily injection of insulin. In cases where the diabetic is capable of producing insulin but only in small amounts, he or she will need to reduce their carbohydrate intake to a quantity that their own insulin supplies can deal with.

If you are persistently plagued with thrush it is important that you be tested for diabetes, especially if there is a history of the disease in your family. The presence of sugar in the urine can indicate diabetes but your doctor should refer you to a hospital for a *full glucose tolerance test*. You will be asked not to eat or drink anything for at least eight hours before the test, which takes about two and a half hours. It's a good idea to take something to read along with you to help to pass the time, and a small snack to eat afterwards. During the test you will be given drinks of glucose. After each drink a sample of your blood will be taken to check the level of glucose. You will be asked for a urine sample before and on completion of the test.

The results of a full glucose tolerance test should come through in about a week. If they are negative and you don't have diabetes the cause of thrush must lie elsewhere.

The vitamin B factor

I was desperate. I tried everything which people advised but the most effective way was my increase in vitamin B6 (pyridoxine). I take 100 milligrams per day and there is no worry of 'over-dosing' as they are water soluble. They will be flushed out of the body if not used. As all my efforts with external applications did not work I thought that attacking the thrush internally would be successful. I have increased my total intake of the B vitamins.

Chapters 2 and 3 dealt with the sort of things which encourage the growth of *Candida*. Some of these should now be discussed again. The contraceptive pill, sugar, diabetes, antibiotics and poor health are relevant here. Why? Because of the link between them and vitamin B6. All of these things increase the body's need for this one particular vitamin. The pill and antibiotics, diabetes, an excessive intake of sugar, and sickness or ill health can cause a deficiency of vitamin B6. And all of them lower the body's resistance to fungal infection. This strongly suggests, therefore, that vitamin B6 is the key to preventing thrush.

The vitamin B family, or vitamin B complex, consists of about eighteen different members. Of these at least twelve can be made chemically. Most of these vitamins are obtained from the same sources so that an inadequate diet will usually be deficient in several of the B vitamins rather than just one of them. Brewer's yeast, wheat-germ and meat are rich in all of the B vitamins. Nuts, beans and lentils, and soya products are other good sources.

Vitamin B1 (thiamin), essential for growth, the conversion of carbohydrates into energy, and the health of the nerves and muscles, is found in most whole-grain foods. Seafood also contains small amounts. Vitamin B2 (riboflavin) which helps to keep the skin, mouth and eyes healthy, is supplied in eggs, vegetables, milk and cheese. Vitamin B6 (pyridoxine) can be obtained from most wholemeal products, oats, milk, fish and cabbage. Liver, meat and eggs provide supplies of vitamin B12 (cyanocobalamine). Choline and insotitol are essential for the functioning of the liver and to prevent the build up of fats in the body. Folic acid is used for making red blood cells. These substances are supplied by offal meats, nuts, green vegetables, yeast and wheatgerm.

A lack of the B vitamins is mainly caused by eating too many refined foods, or over-cooking fresh sources of the vitamins. Like vitamin C they are all water soluble. They dissolve in water just as sugar or salt does. This means that they are easily lost by cooking foods in water. And because they are water soluble they cannot be stored in the body. (Vitamin B12 is an exception. It can be stored in the liver.) If they are not used, any excess will be passed out of the body in the urine. To keep healthy make sure you get a good intake of the B vitamins every day.

A deficiency of vitamin B complex affects the nerves and may result in nervous disorders and depression. These may be indirect causes of thrush. A lack of the B vitamins can result in diseases of the skin. And what is thrush if it is not a skin disease? During illness a person's need for vitamin B increases. Since a vitamin B deficiency makes you prone to thrush, this is why we get attacks when we are poorly, under stress or generally run down.

If you eat too much sugar you are more likely to develop thrush. Women on the pill who eat large amounts of carbo-hydrate may be suffering from attacks, not simply because the fungus thrives on sugar, but also because they are deficient in vitamin B6. A high sugar intake destroys the good bacilli in the intestine and can cause diabetes. Since the B vitamins are water soluble they are readily lost in the urine. Diabetics who excrete large amounts of urine are usually lacking in these vitamins, especially vitamin B6. This is yet another reason why they are so defenceless against thrush.

Certain intestinal bacteria are capable of synthesizing the B vitamins. So, even if your intake of foods containing vitamin B is low, the body may still be producing enough to protect you from thrush. But when these bacteria are destroyed, by antibiotics, for example, or by eating too much sugar, a higher intake of vitamin B will be necessary to prevent fungal growth.

Thrush can be kept at bay by cutting down on sugar *and* increasing your intake of vitamin B. On average we require at least three milligrams of vitamin B1, and from three to five milligrams of vitamin B2 daily. During an attack eat plenty of those foods rich in the B vitamins. Obtain the optimum amount of vitamin B complex as a safeguard against further infections.

> I have been a 'life-longer'. Thrush ebbs and flows with my general state of health but is ever lurking. I once had a long talk with a very understanding (lady) doctor. She seemed to think my lifelong eczema was related to the thrush, especially when I mentioned that I'd been fed copious quantities of vitamin B as a child, and still seemed to need it. She recommended taking vitamin B, either naturally or in concentrated pill form and it does seem to help enormously. It also seems to help PMT, something I was suffering more and more as I got older.

Vitamin B tablets are no real substitute for proper vitamin B rich foods. And if you eat plenty of food containing vitamin B you won't need to take supplementary tablets. Extra vitamin B cannot be stored in the body. It will be excreted in the urine. However, if you aren't getting your maximum quota of vitamin B through your diet it is advisable to take a supplementary dosage in tablet form. These can be brought from most health food stores and chemists.

Yoghurt

Eating live Bulgarian yoghurt is an excellent way of taking vitamin B. It replaces or reinforces the intestinal bacteria which produce this vitamin. All the B vitamins can be synthesized by the bacteria found in yoghurt and/or acidophilus milk. This type of yoghurt can be bought from health food shops but home-made yoghurt is even better. When made with non-instant powdered milk it contains twice the amount of protein, calcium and vitamin B2 that commercially produced yoghurt does. And it's cheaper too!

Thrush

I thoroughly recommend natural yoghurt – it is good for the gut as it repopulates it with the right gut flora, and good for the genitals as it is incredibly soothing. How many foods are so good for one at both ends?

Making your own yoghurt

You will need to buy a tub of live yoghurt or acidophilus culture before you can make your own.

Heat two pints of milk in a saucepan. Bring to the boil and leave to cool until it is only slightly warm. Stir the tub of yoghurt or acidophilus culture into the lukewarm milk. Then pour this into empty cartons, cups or jars and cover. Leave them in a warm place to curdle. (This takes about three to six hours.) The yoghurt must be kept warm so that the bacteria it contains can multiply and sour the milk entirely.

When a thick, firm curd has formed over the milk the yoghurt should be placed in the fridge. This prevents further bacterial growth. It stops the milk from becoming too sour. After about eight hours in the refrigerator the yoghurt should be ready to eat.

More can be made using a part of the yoghurt from your first batch as a new culture. After a month you will probably need to refresh the yoghurt with a more concentrated bought culture.

The importance of a balanced diet cannot be stressed too heavily. Vitamin C (ascorbic acid) is vital in building up the body's resistance to disease. It also helps to prevent allergies. Cabbage, tomatoes and citrus fruits are the richest source of vitamin C, but it is found in all fresh growing fruits and vegetables. Vitamin A (retinol) can be obtained from fish oils, butter and meat. It is necessary to keep the skin and mucous membranes in good condition, and to protect them against all infections. Vitamin A is fat soluble. It can be stored in the body, unlike vitamin C, which must be supplied daily.

I am forty-one years old. I have suffered from thrush for about four years. I got so many attacks that seldom a month passed without it. I got so depressed and tearful last November that I went to talk to a lady doctor at my local Well Woman clinic. She explained what a vicious circle it all was and sent me back to my own doctor. This time, however, he said that he and a colleague had a theory that the iron level in the blood had something to do with women being susceptible to thrush. So I have had a month's course of iron tablets and have not had an attack for four months now.

Minerals, like calcium, phosphorus, iron and iodine, should not be neglected. Amongst their numerous functions they keep the blood and tissue fluids from becoming either too acid or too alkaline. This is of great importance in controlling thrush. Doctors have drawn a link between the incidence of fungal infection and an iron deficiency. Women are more prone to thrush when they become anaemic; that is when they develop a shortage of haemoglobin. Iron is essential because it combines with protein to form haemoglobin. This is the oxygen-carrying component of the red blood cells. Iron allows the blood to function properly. It keeps our tissues healthy. Women are more likely to be deficient in iron than men and are thus more susceptible to anaemia. The average human body contains about three or four grams of iron. Some of this will be lost via the outermost layer of skin, which the body continuously sheds. During menstruation women lose about thirty milligrams each month. In pregnancy the need for iron increases significantly. Liver, meat, eggs and cereals are good sources of this mineral. Most vegetables provide some iron. And the vitamin C that they contain improves the absorption of iron from the intestine.

Acid-forming foods that make the body more acidic reduce the likelihood of getting thrush since the fungus prefers an alkaline environment in which to grow. Most grains, except for millet and buckwheat, are classed as 'acid forming'. They are also particularly rich in the B vitamins too! Fruit juices are highly alkaline. They may encourage thrush to grow, and for this reason should be avoided.

I started with thrush over four years ago and much to my annoyance still have this. Not only do I ruin my underwear, but the irritation of the itchiness, and burning is awful and embarrassing.

I eat plenty of food, and find cheese, coffee and rich food contribute to a certain level of the thrush because, after eating many of these, I find it probably at its worst and the start of it yet again.

To cut a long story short . . . A couple of years ago a friend mentioned a lady doctor who sounded sane, sensible and interested in women's complaints. Off I went to see her. She gave me a long list of foods to cut out of my diet. This was after I had done some research on myself by following and listing the results of a three-week rotating diet. It was hard work but I was determined. Eventually she had me cut out the following foods: cheese – mould forms on it, mushrooms – a fungus, alcohol –made from fermented fruit, yeasty bread – most breads have yeast! I cut them all out and things improved. I have stopped drinking and eating mushrooms and cheese completely. I still have a little bread. Sugar also aggravated the thrush situation for me.

Certain foods tend to precipitate thrush in some women. Cheese seems to be a typical enemy. Alcohol is specially bad, probably because it contains a lot of sugar and because it increases the body's need for vitamin B1. It also inflames the mucous membranes in the intestinal tract. Beer and light wines are less irritating than spirits since their alcohol content is more dilute.

Changing your diet may be *the* change for the better. A thrush problem may be caused or perpetuated by something in your diet. Try not to eat any of the suspect foods like cheese for at least ten days, and see what difference this makes. Should the symptoms of thrush return on resuming your normal diet, it would be wise to avoid these foods permanently. It is possible that your body only reacts to one food in particular. To pinpoint exactly what is causing the trouble, cut out several of the 'baddies' listed in this chapter week by week from your diet. For example, during the first week eliminate sweets and sugary foods. The following week stop eating cheese and so on until the symptoms associated with thrush disappear. If an attack flares up again after an over-indulgence of one of these foods, you will know for certain which one is your enemy!

It is quite likely that many recurrent thrush problems are not related in any way to the sufferer's eating habits. But don't forget that a poor diet invariably leads to poor health, and good health means good riddance to thrush.

EIGHT

About Other Genital Infections

Apart from thrush, there are many other diseases which can affect our sexual and reproductive organs. Most of these are extremely common. They can occur at any time. Some are caused by bacteria. Others are spread by a virus. Some are caught by sexual contact. These are called venereal diseases, and they must be treated immediately.

All of the conditions described in this chapter can cause severe discomfort and emotional distress, especially when they recur. And because the symptoms of so many of these infections can easily be mistaken for thrush, it is very important that all thrush sufferers should know about them.

Trichomonas

This is an infection caused by the parasite, *Trichomonas vaginalis*, a tiny one-celled organism which feeds on other cells. The organism survives in warm, moist environments. In some women it is a normal and harmless inhabitant of the vagina and bladder. When too many of these bugs are present an infection will flare up.

The symptoms of *Trichomonas* can sometimes be confused with thrush. The vagina and vulva become swollen and sore. And there may be tiny red spots on the inner walls of the vagina and cervix. Women with *Trichomonas* will usually notice a thin and foamy discharge, which may be white or greenish-yellow in colour and be excessively smelly. If the urethra and bladder become infected too, there will be a burning sensation when passing urine.

Both men and women suffer from *Trichomonas*, and it can be sexually transmitted – passed from partner to partner during sex. It can also be transferred by hand and so is not confined to heterosexual relationships. *Trichomonas* can survive for a few hours outside the body. Women can become infected from moist towels and wash cloths. Even lavatory seats may harbour the germs for a short while.

It is much easier to detect *Trichomonas* in women since the symptoms are more immediate. The bug can be identified in the urine but the normal procedure carried out at health clinics is to use a 'wet mount'. Some of the vaginal discharge is placed on a glass slide with a saline solution where the *Trichomonads* can be seen swimming about with their whip-like tentacles.

Trichomonas is treated with Flagyl (metronidazole) tablets taken by mouth. Ninety per cent of *Trichomonas* cases are cured in this way. Regular sexual partners must also be treated since they may be infected too. Abstain from sex during treatment to avoid reinfection. Where both partners are being treated simultaneously they may be allowed to continue having sex if a sheath is used.

Flagyl should be used with caution. It is a powerful antibiotic and can actually cause thrush. Women who know themselves to be susceptible to thrush should take appropriate medication concurrently with the Flagyl.

Flagyl also kills off white blood cells. It should not be taken by anyone with blood diseases, or diseases of the central nervous system. It should be taken with food, rather than on an empty stomach. Alcohol should be avoided by anyone taking a course of Flagyl.

Flagyl has some nasty side-effects as well, which include severe nausea, stomach cramps and constipation. Recent studies have shown that Flagyl caused cancer when high dosages were given for a lifetime in some animals. If you have to take more than one course of Flagyl you should wait at least six weeks before beginning the second course. And the manufacturers of the drug, G. D. Searle, recommend a white blood cell count after treatment. Flagyl should never be taken during pregnancy or while breast-feeding, as it can be excreted in the breast milk.

The use of Flagyl alone may not be enough to cure and prevent attacks of *Trichomonas*. Alternative treatments include using chapparral (see Chapter 6) and/or garlic and vinegar remedies. Like thrush, *Trichomonas* prefers less acidic conditions in the vagina and, again like thrush, can be prevented by controlling the pH balance in the genital area. *Trichomonads* prefer blood cells. An attack is likely to be worse during a period. Self-help remedies used around this time are particularly beneficial.

Non-specific vaginitis

Non-specific vaginitis is the name given to an irritated, inflamed or unhealthy vagina. Symptoms of this type of infection include an unusually heavy, white or yellow discharge. Sometimes this is streaked with blood. The vagina may be sore and itchy. There may be a burning sensation on passing urine, and other cystitis-like symptoms.

Although the germs causing the infection are unknown, this type of vaginitis indicates a disturbance of the finely balanced ecology of the vagina. The infection may be brought on by a course of antibiotics, or other drugs, as these tend to reduce the vagina's acidity. In more alkaline conditions bacteria and other organisms – normal inhabitants of the vagina and usually harmless here – rapidly multiply, giving rise to infections. Nylon underwear and tights, harsh soaps and/or vaginal deodorants can cause problems and provoke non-specific vaginitis. This is because these, too, interfere with the acid/alkaline balance of the sex organs. A vagina and vulva irritated from prolonged intercourse are also more susceptible to infection.

Non-specific vaginitis can occur when germs which live happily in *other* parts of the body but *not* in the vagina, find their way here. The rectum, for instance, harbours a great many organisms which can cause problems if they are introduced into the vagina or urethra. Both of these orifices are precariously near to the anus. By wiping towards the vagina, instead of away from it, bacteria from the bowel is easily spread around the vulva. E. coli, a natural inhabitant of the rectum, is one of the main causes of cystitis (see page 17). Urinary infections and non-specific vaginitis can be prevented by always wiping away from the urethra and by washing after passing a stool. Washing before and after sexual activity is also important.

Non-specific vaginitis can be treated. It is best to visit a special clinic where swabs will be taken to try to discover exactly which organism is causing the problem. If the infection is bacterial a sulpha cream like Sultrin or Vagitrol will be prescribed. If no bacteria are found the infection will probably to treated with tetracycline. It is advisable not to have intercourse during treatment and possibly to abstain for a short while afterwards to allow the tissues to heal properly.

Non-specific infections can be remedied using the sort of self-help measures outlined in Chapter 6. These may also help to prevent recurrences. Garlic, with its antibiotic properties, can be effective in treating bacterial vaginitis. Insert a peeled clove into the vagina every morning for a week, removing the old clove before inserting a new one.

A non-specific infection may also respond to vinegar and salt water solutions. Doctors tend to recommend salt baths for women who suffer from vaginitis a lot. But before you dash off to the bathroom, remember that frequent bathing can sometimes do more harm than good, and can possibly provoke an attack of thrush.

Gardnerella vaginalis

Gardnerella, or *Hemophilius*, is a strain of bacteria which has only recently been discovered as a cause of vaginitis. It is an infection of the vaginal secretions rather than of the vaginal walls. But, like most vaginitis, it occurs when the vagina's delicate flora is upset. Present in every healthy vagina, *Gardnerella* is only troublesome if conditions here become too alkaline. Like thrush, *Gardnerella* is very itchy. It produces a creamy white or grey vaginal discharge. This is often frothy. So it is not uncommon for doctors to mistake *Gardnerella* for *Trichomonas* or thrush.

The condition can be diagnosed at a special clinic. Unfortunately, the usual treatment available is a course of Flagyl (see page 64), which can trigger off an attack of thrush. Women with *Gardnerella* who are prone to fungal infections should always ask for a course of thrush treatment to take concurrently with the Flagyl.

Some clinics prefer to treat *Gardnerella* with sulpha creams and/or pessaries. Tetracycline is prescribed for the infected male partner. To prevent reinfection both partners *must* be treated.

A combined garlic and vinegar solution (see Chapter 6)

may be used as an alternative treatment. Inserting acidophilus capsules into the vagina after each treatment with
the solution to restore the vagina's natural acidity will help
to prevent the condition recurring.

Atrophic vaginitis

This is not an infection in the truest sense of the word since
it is not caused by a germ. It is often a plague on women's
sexual health, however, and can be an indirect cause of
thrush and other vaginal infections.

Atrophic vaginitis is an inflammation which occurs
when the vaginal walls do not produce enough lubricating
mucus. It is normally associated with the menopause when
the decrease in a woman's oestrogen level causes the walls
of the vagina to lose much of their moisture and elasticity.
The vagina then becomes more exposed to infection. Intercourse may be painful and the tender mucous membranes
of the vagina are easily bruised and/or torn.

This condition can be treated with oestrogen creams
applied directly to the vagina. A simple lubricating cream,
like KY Jelly, which can be bought over the counter at a
chemist's, will also help, particularly during intercourse.

Vaginismus

Like atrophic vaginitis this is not an infection. Vaginismus
is a medical term referring to a *spasm*, or contraction of the
muscles around the vagina, which makes intercourse difficult or impossible and very painful.

The cause of vaginismus may be a physical one. An
unstretched hymen will make penetration difficult and
painful. If penetration is attempted when a woman is in-
sufficiently sexually aroused the vagina may be too dry to
accept her partner's penis. Perhaps, more importantly, are
the emotional reasons which bring about vaginismus. The
involuntary contraction of the vaginal muscles may be an
unconscious protest against sex. Suffering with a vaginal
infection such as thrush, even for a short while, under-
mines a woman's confidence in her own body. One of the
most distressing aspects of sexual ill-health is that it makes

the sufferer feel inhibited about making love. Learning to relax will help your vaginal muscles to relax, and thus make sex less painful and more enjoyable. But if you suspect that vaginismus may be caused by a physical reason, visit your doctor.

Non-infective leukorrhoea

Healthy organs and tissues are made up of millions of cells and the vagina, or course, is no exception. Throughout our lives it is constantly replacing these cells – as old ones die, new ones are formed. The old dead cells are passed out of the body, unnoticed, with the usual vaginal secretions. The term 'non-infective leukorrhoea' refers to a heavy discharge which occurs when too many of these cells are being broken down. This discharge is usually white – so that it can be mistaken for thrush – and may be irritating. The increased amount of vaginal fluid may attract bacteria. Stale secretions around the vulva and in your pants will increase the likelihood of infection. Washing the genital area at least once a day with cool, plain water will minimize the irritation – but remember that a heavy vaginal discharge invariably signals a problem. It is always best to visit a doctor if the symptoms persist and/or the condition worsens. Non-infective leukorrhoea is more common in older women.

Cervicitis and cervical erosion

Cervicitis means an inflammation or infection on or around the cervix. Many women suffer from this complaint without knowing about it. They only find out after an internal examination or because they have another infection like thrush. Others experience a heavy discharge – white or yellow in colour, and possibly streaked with blood, or cystitis–like symptoms when the infection begins to affect the urethra.

The term 'cervical erosion' is ambiguous. Most doctors use the word as a blanket term to describe a red or inflamed patch on the cervix. *Cervical eversion* is frequently diagnosed as *erosion*.

The cervix is made up of two basic types of cells. The outer lining of the cervix is composed of pink cells. These are called *squamous cells*. Cervical eversion means that the soft red *columnar cells* from inside the cervix have spread on to the outer cervix, pushing the *squamous cells* aside. The columnar cells are very sensitive. They are highly susceptible to infection and can be bruised or damaged during intercourse. An *erosion* occurs when the cervix has actually been damaged and has lost some of its surface cells. It is rather like a graze. An *eroded* cervix looks red and sore because the delicate tissues normally protected by the squamous cells are exposed. Bleeding after sex, and/or bleeding between periods are signs of cervical erosion. An erosion/eversion or cervicitis may be aggravating a persistent or recurring thrush problem. For this reason all three conditions need to be treated as soon as possible.

Cervicitis is treated in much the same way as non-specific vaginitis – with sulpha creams or pessaries and/or antibiotics (e.g. tetracycline). An erosion or eversion can be successfully dealt with in one or two ways: by cauterising the cervix, burning off the layer of cells, or with cryo-surgery, where the cells are frozen. Some doctors prefer to leave an erosion alone particularly if it is neither trouble-some nor infected. However, if you continually suffer from infections like thrush or non-specific vaginitis, any disorder of the cervix must be seen to.

Cervical cancer

Cancer of the cervix is the most common of the cancers specific to women. Fortunately, it can be diagnosed at an early stage where the growth and spread of the cancer can be prevented.

Cervical cancer is detected by carrying out a smear test. This is simple and painless. The cervix is gently scraped with a wooden spatula. The cells from the scraping are then examined under a microscope.

The results of the test will either be positive or negative. A positive smear does not mean that you have cancer. It simply shows that some of the cells are changing. The stages of cervical cancer are part of a continuum and the theory is that the changing cells can progress through the early stages to invasive cancer. This is still not fully understood, since, even without treatment, the cell changes may stop at any stage, and even return to normal. And the speed at which the cancer develops varies greatly.

It is quite common for women to have abnormal smears. The majority of positive results indicate an infection or irritation of the cervix. An eversion would almost definitely result as a positive smear. Anyone with a positive result would be asked to return for a follow-up test, and for repeat smears every six or twelve months. Doctors in Britain are only paid to give cervical smears to women over thirty-five, and to women who have had three or more children. But special clinics and family planning clinics carry out these tests as a matter of routine. Any heterosexually active woman should be screened at least once a year.

The exact reasons why cancer of the cervix develops are not known. Doctors think that there is a link between the cancer and sexual promiscuity. But how many sexual partners must a woman have before she can be labelled as promiscuous? And what about the promiscuous male? It would seem that monogamous women whose partners frequently have extra-marital sex are equally at risk.

How can cervical cancer be avoided? Barrier methods of contraception may help – they are known to be good protection against VD. But the most effective way of preventing cervical cancer is by making sure that regular smear tests are carried out throughout a woman's lifetime.

Herpes

Herpes are cold sores, which look like blisters or small bumps. They may appear on the thighs, in or near the anus, or on the buttocks. In women, herpes sores are typically found in and around the vagina, on the vulva and on the cervix. They are caused by the virus, *Herpes simplex 2*, similar to the type which produces cold sores or blisters around the mouth and nose. Herpes are nearly always transmitted sexually.

This is a most distressing complaint. The sores are

normally extremely painful, especially if they rupture. Open sores are highly infectious. And they are, themselves, subject to infection from other bacteria. It may take anything from a week to one month for an attack to clear up. When the sores disappear the virus enters a latent stage, when it is no longer contagious. A new attack can occur at any time. There is no limit to the number of attacks a herpes sufferer may experience, although for many people the first attack is the worst.

As yet there is no known cure for herpes. The symptoms can be relieved with sulpha creams and corticosteroids. Wearing loose cotton clothing and underwear during an attack helps. Try to keep the area cool and dry.

It has been suggested that there is a strong link between herpes and cancer of the cervix. For this reason women who suffer from herpes should have frequent cervical smear tests, preferably every six to twelve months.

Warts

Genital warts, like ordinary warts, are caused by a virus which may lie dormant for up to three months or more. They are infectious and are sexually transmitted although they may be spread in other ways. They tend to grow more readily in warm and moist areas of the body. Women with a heavy vaginal discharge are more likely to develop warts, where they appear inside or outside the vagina or around the anus.

Warts can be felt as hard lumps but they are rarely painful. In spite of this anyone with warts should get them removed since they can be passed on to sexual partners.

Special clinics and doctors will treat warts. Small warts can be frozen off (cryosurgery). Usually, however, warts are burnt off with a weekly painting of podophyllum solution. The treatment must be continued until all the warts have disappeared. Any that are left will only spread again. And, as with all genital infections, sexual partners must be treated too.

Crab lice

Intense itching around the genitals might be caused by crab lice which infest the pubic hair. Like other types of lice, crabs are bloodsuckers. They attach themselves to the hair, close to the roots, where they bite into the skin. They quickly lay their eggs – or nits – which stick to the hair until they hatch several days later. This type of lice prefer coarse, wiry hair. They infest the pubic hair but occasionally may be found in the hair on the chest, armpits, eyelashes and eyebrows.

Crab lice are usually transferred during intercourse but they may be acquired through other kinds of close personal contact. It is possible to catch crabs by sleeping in the same bed as an infected person, or from contaminated bedding and towels.

Normal soap doesn't affect lice. They are easily destroyed, however, with special shampoos, cream or powder which can be bought from a chemist's, or obtained free from a special clinic. Have a bath and dry yourself thoroughly before applying the lotion. Leave on for twenty-four hours before washing it off. Away from the body, crabs die within a day but the nits can survive for six days. Because of this, clothing, sheets and blankets should be boiled or dry cleaned, or left for a week before they are used again.

Gonorrhoea

Gonorrhoea is an infection of the genito-urinary organs. It is only transmitted sexually – through intercourse or intimate contact with an infected person. This is because the bacterium which causes the disease – the gonoccocus – cannot survive for any length of time away from the body. The gonoccocus thrives in warm, moist environments. The organisms are transferred when natural moisture or discharge from an infectious person is deposited on the genitals of another sexual partner during intercourse. It is possible to develop gonorrhoea in the throat if oral/genital contact takes place. Occasionally sufferers may infect their own eyes.

Gonorrhoea is more dangerous than any of the complaints that have been discussed in this chapter. Left untreated it can have serious complications and cause sterility.

Women with gonorrhoea rarely show any symptoms until its irreparable damage has been done. There may be a vaginal discharge, and some discomfort on passing water. But for most women these symptoms are so mild as to be unnoticeable. In the majority of cases women are not aware that they have gonorrhoea unless they are told by an infected male partner.

Except in very rare circumstances men develop symptoms, usually some two to five days after contracting gonorrhoea. At first, there is a burning sensation on passing urine. This is then followed by a penile discharge of yellow pus as the disease begins to affect the urethra. In women, the most common site of early uncomplicated gonorrhoea is the cervix. There may be a cervical discharge. The urethra may also be affected. But even in cases where both the urethra and cervix are involved, there may still be no warning signs of infection.

Sometimes small abscesses form around the external opening of the urethra. When the inflammation spreads along the urethra to the base of the bladder, it will cause cystitis-like symptoms. Sufferers will experience a frequent urge to urinate although there may be only a small amount of water to pass. What little there is burns very badly.

Vaginal gonorrhoea may easily spread to the rectum since, in women, the vaginal and anal orifices are so close to one another. Infected discharge seeps into the anus causing *proctitis* – or inflammation of the rectum. There may be few visible signs of anal-rectal gonorrhoea. However, some women do develop a slight anal discharge, more noticeable in the stools.

The early complications of gonorrhoea are severe but they can be treated effectively. Without proper medical attention the harm done to a woman's internal organs is often irremediable. The disease spreads up the cervical canal, through the uterus, to the Fallopian tubes – the tubes that 'carry' eggs from the ovaries to the womb. When the Fallopian tubes become inflamed, this is called *salpingitis*. You may have pain on one or both sides of the lower abdomen, accompanied by vomiting and/or fever. If the infection is allowed to progress further, the Fallopian tubes become twisted with scar tissue. This can result in complete sterility once the tubes become blocked.

Gonorrhoea must be treated at a VD or special clinic (see pages 31–34). These clinics offer the best facilities for the accurate diagnosis of all genital infections. Gonorrhoea is particularly difficult to detect in women. Discharge or a scraping from the cervix, rectum and urethra will be microscopically examined. Cultures of the gonoccocus will be made in the laboratory. Sometimes a blood sample will be taken and tested for gonorrhoea.

Treatment is usually with a large dose of penicillin. This is given by injection, and ensures the greatest percentage of cures in a large number of patients. When penicillin cannot be given – for example, when a patient is allergic to the drug – one of the tetracycline group of antibiotics will be prescribed. Patients will be asked not to have sex and to refrain from alcohol until they are completely free of infection.

Because gonorrhoea is so damaging for women it is imperative to return for follow-up examinations. Repeated examinations and tests after treatment are essential since it is as difficult to establish whether the condition has been cured in women as it is to detect it in the first place. Remember that it is crucial to get prompt medical attention at the first signs of *any* vaginal infection. (A vaginal discharge from gonorrhoea can easily be mistaken for other types of vaginitis.) And if you think that you might have been exposed to the infection – even if you don't have any symptoms at all – go to a special clinic and ask to be checked out.

NINE

Sex

Although I am now thrush-free, I am an extremely frigid woman. I find it very difficult to make love with my husband although I force myself to and hope and pray that by forcing myself I will one day return to my former self, enjoying a perfectly natural and happy sexual relationship with my husband. I am also very sure that he suspects my frigidity – I certainly hope not – but how is it possible to hide one's true feelings from the one you love?

A permanent battle against a recurring vaginal infection devalues a woman's sexual worth, and her self-esteem. All too often when a problem affects our sex lives, sex itself becomes a problem too. Thrush is irritating, painful and demoralizing. But the psychological effects it leaves behind even if, and when, the infection finally resolves itself are often the hardest to accept.

Sexual problems invariably inflict considerable pressure on any sexual relationship. And being unable to make love because of a scourge like thrush can be very frustrating indeed! Women who suffer a lot from vaginal infections need understanding and sympathetic lovers and husbands. Enormous amounts of patience and tolerance are required of both partners if the relationship is to survive the weeks of celibacy which make such heavy demands upon it.

Emotional stress complicates the problem. The lower you feel, the more vulnerable you are to the infection. It's another vicious circle.

I have found sex to be the great aggravator and it all starts off again. Unless a course of pessaries are followed for about a month then they don't work and it's difficult to abstain for that long, or I start to get problems with the relationship, feel un-feminine and can't stand anyone near. It's an endless cycle of misery!

Thrush has serious repercussions in other ways. Women

who suffer from vaginal infections may feel inhibited and unconfident about making love, especially about oral/genital contact. One or both partners in a sexual relationship may be unwilling to have intercourse for fear of provoking further attacks.

> At present, I honestly don't know whether I have thrush still or not. I am keeping my fingers crossed and hoping I can forget the fear of it returning since psychologically I feel the pain of intercourse, caused by thrush, has made me wary of resuming sexual relations.

It is sometimes difficult to decide whether or not a thrush problem is related to sex. For many women it seems to make little difference. Thrush makes its presence felt, month after month, sex or no sex. It is generally advisable, however, not to have sex if you are feeling the slightest hint of vaginal discomfort. Tears and abrasions in the mucous membranes of the vaginal walls are an excellent breeding ground for bacteria which normally live (and die) without causing problems around a healthy vulva.

The chances of permanent relief from thrush rest on a good relationship between doctor and patient. Never allow a doctor to tell you to 'give up sex for a while'. Self-imposed celibacy is *not* a cure for thrush. Such comments are meaningless – how long is 'a while' anyway? Nor does it resolve thrush since it tends to imply that as soon as sex is resumed the problem will return.

Providing that an attack of thrush has cleared up properly, and that the tissues have been given time to heal, sexual intercourse should not be painful. It is quite normal to feel a little soreness after sex. But an inflamed, swollen or itchy vulva would suggest that the condition has either recurred or has never been effectively cleared up.

> I used to dread having sex, because it would hurt so much and because I would invariably develop thrush afterwards. I was so tense that I could never enjoy love making. I went to my doctor who said I was suffering from 'vaginismus' and this was probably the cause of my thrush. Although my problem was an emotional one, it could be treated physically. The doctor told me that learning to relax the vaginal muscles is particularly important

in preventing and curing vaginal infections. Exercising these muscles stimulates and increases the blood supply to the genitals. And when you increase the blood flow it means that more white blood cells reach the vagina to keep the area healthy.

During an attack

Never have intercourse during an attack of vaginal thrush as this will increase your discomfort. It may also prolong the infection. Thrush is sexually transmissible. It can be passed from partner to partner during sex. The chances of becoming reinfected are much higher if sex takes place again before the condition has been cleared. Men rarely show any signs of the infection although they may be carrying thrush spores. Unless both partners are treated for thrush it is likely that as soon as sexual contact resumes, thrush will recur.

When both partners of a sexual relationship are being treated for thrush simultaneously some doctors see no reason for lovemaking to cease. Bearing in mind how tender a vagina inflamed by *Candida* will be, it is sensible to forgo this sort of advice. Abstaining from sex for a short period of time allows the delicate tissues around the surface sex organs to heal themselves and will lessen the likelihood of the thrush returning.

Don't be tempted, therefore! Don't have sexual intercourse while you are being treated for thrush. This may be some time. But it is better to wait than to carry on as normal, only to see the infection flare up time and time again.

Here are a few rules about sex which, if they are followed every time you make love, should help to prevent recurrences of thrush and similar types of vaginitis:

1. Only have sex when it feels all right, and don't have sex during an attack of thrush even if it is painless.

2. It is good practice to wash before and after intercourse. This helps to wash away bacteria and prevent infection. Pouring cold water over the vulva and perineum after sex reduces the swelling or bruising that may have been incurred during sex. This also helps to prevent urinary

infections like cystitis because it washes germs away from the urethra.

3. Go to the lavatory *immediately* after sex to flush away bacteria from the urethra. Again, this is particularly important in the prevention of cystitis.

4. Until you are certain that an attack of thrush has been cleared up, avoid oral/genital sex. Remember that it is possible to develop thrush in the mouth.

5. Many women are more prone to thrush at certain stages in their monthly cycle. Avoiding intercourse at this time reduces the chances of another attack if the condition is aggravated by sex. For example, if thrush tends to recur just after a period, don't have sex during the period, and refrain for a few days afterwards until the 'danger time' has passed.

6. Always use a sterile, water-soluble lubricant, such as KY Jelly during sex if you need to.

> Thrush! Such an irritating problem in more ways than one. I've suffered with it for eleven years since the birth of my first daughter. I found intercourse impossible while suffering and of course totally useless as it only made matters worse. I seem to start with thrush on most occasions when intercourse has occurred without good lubrication. So I make sure I've always my KY Jelly at hand.

On a final note, it is worth remembering that the use of spermicidal creams or foams can be the source of a persistent vaginal infection. These contain powerful chemicals. They can irritate the mucous membranes of the vagina and vulva. They may also affect the delicate pH balance of the vagina. Some women are allergic to spermicides and should not use them.

Using a barrier method of contraception helps to reduce the chances of reinfection. It is known that sheaths are a good barrier against VD, and there's no reason why this shouldn't apply to thrush.

> I suffered for three months with persistent thrush and throughout this time abstained from sex. The hardest thing of all for me

was resuming sexual relations with my boyfriend. At each attempt I was incredibly tense and convinced that any touching of my genitals was going to be extremely painful, which made love-making impossible and the thought of penetration unbearable. This was such an ironical situation as, although I was thrush-free, I still could not make love.

However, through working in a hospital, I managed to see a gynaecologist. He showed nothing but kindness and understanding . . . and was very concerned that I should resume my happy sex life. He prescribed Aci-jel which, although it is quite messy, worked wonders because it supplied copious amounts of lubrication. The first time I was still apprehensive, but gradually I regained my confidence.

TEN

A Way of Life

Many doctors are becoming aware of self-help and preventative measures as treatments for thrush. In the past women have often had to resign themselves to a lifetime of vaginal discomfort, celibacy and extreme misery. Today, learning to live with thrush is absurd. Learning to prevent it makes sense!

Out of sight, out of mind

Getting to know your vagina is the best way to prevent vaginal infections and to protect yourself against thrush. Few of us bother to examine our bodies very often, though the importance of regular self-examination cannot be stressed too strongly. Because our sexual organs are safely concealed between our legs they generally tend to be ignored. Surprisingly enough, it is possible for any woman to get a glimpse of her vagina and cervix, though she will rarely be advised to do so.

It is important to look at the external genitals so that the warning signs of a vaginal infection can be detected at the earliest opportunity. Most vaginal infections begin high up in the vaginal canal. By the time they hit the surface sex organs and become symptomatic, preventative medicine will have little or no effect. It is wise, therefore, to include internal examinations as part of your self-help programme. Doing so will help you to spot vaginal irritations, like thrush, before they become a big problem.

A do-it yourself internal examination

Before you begin you will need a speculum. This is a device used by doctors to separate the walls of the vagina so that they can get a clear view of the membranes lining the vagina and cervix. You can buy a plastic speculum from a surgical appliance store. Or ask for one at a special clinic or at a family planning clinic.

Plastic speculum

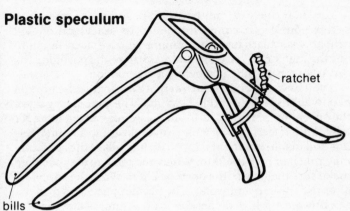

ratchet

bills

You will also need a mirror and a strong light. Use a directional lamp or a powerful torch. A non-greasy, water-soluble lubricant such as KY Jelly will help you to insert the speculum more easily.

Lie down on a couch or on the floor. Make sure that you are comfortable. Use a couple of pillows or cushions to support your head and shoulders. Insert the speculum side-ways into the vagina, pushing it downwards and slightly backwards towards the small of your back. When it is fully in, turn the speculum so that the handles are pointing upwards. Slowly pull the handles together. This opens the bills of the speculum and holds the vaginal walls apart. You don't usually have to open a speculum as wide as it will go. The second or third notch along the ratchet should be wide enough. It is a good idea to practise opening and closing the speculum before you put it inside you.

Direct the light at the mirror and you will be able to see into the dark passage – your vagina. The vaginal walls will look very much like the lining of your throat. At the end of the vagina is the cervix, the base or neck of the uterus. You will notice a dimple in the cervix. This is called the os. It is the actual opening of the cervix into the womb, through which the menstrual flow passes.

You may have to adjust or re-position the speculum before your cervix comes into view. Its exact location will probably vary each time you examine yourself since, throughout the menstrual cycle, the uterus changes its position. The cervix lowers slightly just before menstruation.

If you have never done an internal examination before you may want to get a friend to help you. The vagina may reject the speculum at first so re-insert it carefully, using more KY Jelly, until it feels comfortable. Never close a speculum while it is still inside the vagina. If you do the bills of the speculum may pinch or nick the skin. When you remove the speculum make sure that it is in the open position. Wash the speculum after use in soap and water. The plastic speculums that you can buy are marked 'disposable' but, as long as they are kept clean, they can be used again and again. It is best to sterilize a speculum if you use it during a yeast infection. But don't boil a plastic speculum – it will melt!

What you will see

The walls of the vagina are usually palish pink. If they appear to be puffy or red, this is a sign of inflammation and should not be ignored. A heavy white discharge indicates some sort of vaginal infection – probably, but not always, *Candida*. And if the vaginal walls are white it is very likely that you've got thrush. The white fungus might also collect around the external labia and in the folds of the clitoris.

It is normal to have a slight discharge. The membranes that line the vagina and the glands of the cervix secrete moisture and mucus. This moisture is usually transparent or milky-white, and slippery. The amount and consistency of this discharge will vary throughout the month. For most women it is slightly heavier at ovulation (about the middle of the menstrual cycle) or before a period. The secretions from the vagina increase when we are sexually aroused and during pregnancy. And the amount of vaginal secretion will also depend on a woman's personal hormone balance.

Have a good look at the vulva too. The outer lips, or labia majora, are soft and thick. They may be covered with pubic hair. The inner lips or labia minora protect the vaginal and urethral openings. The labia will vary in colour, from pale pink to dark brown. When we are sexually aroused they swell and turn darker. Generally speaking, in its normal unexcited state, a vibrant red, swollen or inflamed vulva is an indication of a vaginal infection. And it will probably feel as sore as it looks.

These broad guidelines should not be read as hard and fast rules. Remember that what is normal varies just as much as one woman's body varies from another. The best way to know what is normal for you is to keep a check on the vagina. This way you will easily be able to detect any abnormality. Keep a note of what you look and feel like when you don't have thrush, as well as when you do have it. You may forget what your vagina and vulva should feel like in their normal state, particularly after you have been suffering from thrush for a long time. Don't put up with vaginal discomfort. Remember that it is not normal to be in pain. A normal vaginal discharge is not offensive. It shouldn't itch or sting. Never assume that an unnatural discharge or irritation indicates yet another attack of thrush as they could be symptoms of a very different type of infection.

Soreness or dryness, a strong smelling, dark-coloured or frothy discharge, itching or burning, or sore spots on or around the genitals are warning signs of possible infection. Symptoms like these could indicate a multitude of complaints. If you are in doubt, visit your doctor.

After a while you should be able to spot an attack of thrush before it has properly begun. How often should you examine yourself? At first, inspect yourself every day – if this is possible. In this way you will familiarize yourself with the numerous changes that occur throughout the menstrual cycle. And you will build up a clear picture of what is normal for you at each stage.

Thereafter, examine yourself regularly – every week or so, for example, and at once if you notice an itch or twinge in the genital area. Conscious care of the vagina and vulva is your safeguard against disease.

Self-protection against thrush

It is good practice to follow these simple preventative measures and to keep to them at all times, as far as this is possible. Some of these have been discussed in Chapters 2 and 3. They are mentioned again because they are so very important if we are to keep thrush at bay.

Keeping cool

Thrush is exacerbated by warmth. This is why thrush sufferers generally experience their worst attacks during the summer. And the itching and discomfort associated with the condition are likely to be more severe at night when you are tucked up in a warm bed. Making sure that the vulva is cool and well ventilated will help to keep thrush in abeyance.

The weave of nylon and synthetic fabrics is impervious to normal circulating air. It is too closely knit to allow fresh air to pass through it. Nylon pants retain heat from the body. They won't absorb the natural daily secretions from the vagina. This discharge will collect around the vulva. In no time at all the crotch can become a very hot and sticky place. Such humid conditions provide an ideal breeding ground for thrush. Fresh cold air destroys fungus spores. Nylon pants encourage their growth. Always make sure that you wear only undies made from 100 per cent cotton. Change your underwear every day. Wearing no pants at all is a good idea, especially when you are recovering from a vaginal infection.

If you live in jeans then it's time to change your wardrobe! Tight trousers are a health hazard. They can actually cause thrush. And they certainly won't make an existing attack any better. They may also be responsible for recurrent thrush. Heavy denim jeans rub together when you walk. This causes friction. Friction generates heat. And heat, of course, means trouble. Wear loose-fitting cotton trousers instead. Providing that they are comfortable – to walk and sit around in – they shouldn't cause you any problems.

I control my attacks by never wearing slacks, tight panties and anything made with man-made fibres. My tights have been converted into stockings with a pair of scissors. I have never connected attacks of *Candida* with either food or drink – only with heat and lack of ventilation between the legs, and man-made fibrous materials.

Don't wear tights if you suffer from thrush. Instead, wear stockings or suspender tights with an open gusset. Pretty Polly do a range of these. Tytex tights are ingenious one-legged 'tights'. They may be more comfortable than ordinary stockings. They are economical too. You don't have to throw both 'legs' away when only one of them is laddered. Both brands should be obtainable from large department stores. Nylon trousers must also be avoided. Ski pants may be very trendy but they are not conducive to good health. At work many women have to wear nylon trousers as part of a uniform. Try to explain to your employer what happens when you are encased in layers of nylon all day long. Ask for a similar pair of cotton trousers to wear instead. It is just possible that the management aren't aware of the effect nylon can have on a woman's body!

In recent years the craze for keep-fit has increased tremendously. And tight-fitting lycra sports wear has become a fashion in its own right. Footless tights and leotards are a lethal combination to exercise in. Nylon and other synthetic fabrics are non-absorbent and impervious to air. After a session in the gym the body is bound to become very sweaty. An attack of thrush can develop within minutes under such humid conditions.

> The main condition, I felt, that caused thrush to recur was when I got hot and sweaty, i.e. when playing sport – which I do a lot, or did, especially at school, and you discover that under your arms aren't the only places that get damp! I began to change my attire when doing strenuous sport or keep fit. I wore cotton running shorts and vests instead of these flashy nylon leotards and tights which thrush absolutely adores. I ensured that I had a shower straight after any exercises at sports halls or failing that, as soon as I got home. A surprising amount of people do not do this.

Hygiene

Keeping the genital area clean and fresh is the best protection against infection. Wash the vulva about once a day. This should be sufficient to keep the vagina healthy and odour-free, and will prevent the build-up of stale vaginal secretions. The easiest way to wash yourself is to pour cool, pure water over the vulva. You can do this squatting in the bath – use a shower attachment if you have one – or while you sit on the lavatory. Use a little plain soap around the anus. Part your legs and pour more water over the vulva and anus. Make sure that you rinse off all the soap. In very hot weather pouring cold water over the surface sex organs will help to cool down a sweaty crotch and safeguard you against thrush.

Try to avoid baths and take showers instead. If you don't have a shower, crouching in the bath, pouring mugfuls of warm water over your body, will keep you as clean as any long hot soak, and is kinder to your vagina. But if you must have baths, bathe in shallow water. The temperature should be lukewarm or cool. Try not to soak for more than a few minutes each time. Baths aren't very good for you but they are far worse when you add strongly scented bath oils or foams to the water. Antiseptics and disinfectants are just as bad. Always make sure that the bath is clean before you put yourself into it! Traces of scouring powder and bath cleansers in the water can destroy the vaginal bacteria which help to ward off infections like thrush. Sitting in a bidet or a bowl of water is quite dangerous. The water provides an ideal medium in which germs can work their way around the vulva and it is possible to wash thrush spores from the anus into the vagina. Some women prefer to wash themselves with a flannel. This is a practice which should be avoided. Such cloths only harbour germs unless they are boiled each time they are used. Dirty flannels may be a constant source of reinfection for thrush sufferers.

Always wash your bottom after every bowel movement. Wipe yourself from front to back, wiping germs away from the vagina and urethral opening. Thrush isn't the only germ that lurks in the bowel. E coli is a natural inhabitant here, and can cause endless misery when it finds its way into the urethra, as the hundreds of women suffering from cystitis will know. Toilet paper alone isn't enough to stop destructive germs from spreading around the genitals. Thrush spores from the bowel must be washed away before they get on to your pants and work their way up to the vagina and urethra. If it isn't possible to have a 'proper wash' after passing a stool, wiping the anus with damp wads of toilet paper or tissues will suffice as an emergency measure. Pat yourself dry with more tissues or toilet paper.

Overwashing is a problem in itself since this may disturb the natural biological defences of the vagina. Don't be too fastidious about hygiene and cleanliness. Remember that it is always possible to wash more germs into the vagina than you are actually washing out.

Washing your clothes

Washing should complement personal hygiene. Washing powder is a skin irritant. Biological detergents are more dangerous. The skin may develop an allergic reaction to the harsh chemicals they contain. The mucous membranes around the genitals are extremely sensitive. The way you wash your clothes can be significantly influential in preventing vaginal inflammation and infection.

Boiling underwear in plain water is the best way to wash your pants. There is no need to add soap. The high temperatures will destroy bacteria and fungus. Keep a special pan aside for this purpose. Alternatively, put your pants into a bowl or sink and pour boiling water over them. Leave to soak for about five minutes and then wash in the usual way.

During an attack of thrush your underwear will have been contaminated by a lot of thrush spores, so that boiling is particularly important. To avoid re-infection run a very hot iron over the gusset. This should remove any remaining traces of *Candida*.

Holidays

We all deserve a holiday every now and then. A change is as good as a rest – or so it is said. Even a short break can be a marvellous tonic. A chance to forget about thrush and really enjoy yourself! Ironically, holidays are often a nightmare for thrush sufferers. An abrupt change in climate and diet may spark off an attack regardless of whether you have managed to keep thrush-free for quite some time. Suddenly all the weeks of hard work, rigidly adhering to the 'dos' and 'don'ts' of a self-help routine, seem to be wasted.

Travelling for several hours in a hot and sweaty car or bus, stuck to a plastic seat, dripping with perspiration, is one of the quickest ways to develop an attack of thrush. When you sit for long periods of time in the same position, air can't circulate around the vulva. Stale sweat and vaginal moisture will begin to accumulate between your thighs. Add 'heat' to this moisture and you create an excellent environment for thrush. Before you go on holiday make sure that the clothes you intend to travel in are comfortable and loose. Don't travel in tights or tight trousers or you will be inviting trouble. At each stop along your journey, get out and walk about. Let some fresh air reach your perineum.

Thrush might start up on holiday, either if it is too hot and you haven't taken suitable clothing with you, or because of poor or limited washing facilities around you. It's pretty difficult to keep clean when you are camping on a desolate moor or hillside! Another reason why we get attacks is that holidays by the sea tend to mean a lot of time is spent in water. Frequent dips in the sea or swimming pool are as bad for your body as long, hot baths. Swimming pools are much worse because of the chlorine added to the water. Chlorine is a powerful germ-killer. It will destroy the bacilli that inhabit the vagina, and leave it open to invading thrush spores. You can minimize the effects of chlorine by rinsing yourself with plain water after each dip in the pool. If it is possible take a shower, but pouring pure water over the vulva will ensure that at least some of the chlorine is washed out of the vagina.

Change out of a damp bikini or swimming costume as soon as you can. Salt and sand will adhere to the damp material. They will chafe the tender skin around the surface sex organs. Pat yourself dry with a soft towel. Use a little talcum powder around the tops of your legs if you're still a bit wet there. And always allow a swimming costume to dry out thoroughly between wearings. Otherwise fungus spores might grow in the gusset.

On holiday try not to relax the rules about sex. Wash before and after intercourse. Use lots of KY Jelly too, or Aci-jel if you have some. These will help to keep the vagina sufficiently lubricated to prevent nicks in the vaginal walls, and will ward off vaginal infections. Aci-jel is especially good. It lets you have fun and maintains the vagina's acidity at the same time.

Don't be slack about your diet. It may be difficult to say no to foreign food. Anything that you are served in a restaurant, or buy from a take-away is liable to be high in calories and probably in carbohydrate as well. Most foreign dishes are very rich and spicy. They may provoke a full scale attack of thrush.

On the continent, the local wine will be flowing freely. Be careful if alcohol has been responsible for many thrush attacks in the past. Too much alcohol can also cause cystitis. Alcohol is a diuretic – that is, it excites the kidneys into producing urine. It is also a bladder irritant. If you are prone to urinary infections, alcohol can be more trouble than it is worth. A holiday with thrush and/or cystitis won't be much fun. Try to drink lots of plain water during the day, especially if the weather is hot. Under a powerful sun, large quantities of the body's fluid will be lost through sweat. To prevent yourself from becoming dehydrated, drink plenty of non-alcoholic liquid. This will also help to negate the effects of a little alcohol in the evenings. Buy bottled water to drink, and to wash with, if the water on tap looks slightly suspect.

The best way to avoid thrush on holiday is to have a vaginal check-up before you go. You can do this yourself, using the self-examination method described at the beginning of this chapter. Alternatively, visit your local special clinic, Well Woman clinic or health centre. If the doctor can't spot anything, and you feel fine, you will probably be all right on holiday. But remember that an attack can strike at any time. It's better to take too many emergency supplies on holiday with you, than to suffer in agony until you arrive home and can get treatment. The thrush sufferer's motto should always be 'be prepared!'.

Here is a list of things to take with you in case of emergencies:

- A mild lanolin cream, to 'block' the infection.

- A small bottle or plastic container of witch hazel.

- Some cotton wool.

- KY Jelly.
- Aci-jel therapeutic vaginal jelly.
- Tampons and/or minipads.

You will need a 'blocking' cream if an attack of thrush develops and you are unable to get to a health clinic. It will relieve the itching and shouldn't mask the symptoms when you finally manage to locate a doctor. Apply witch hazel to the external labia with swabs of cotton wool. This will soothe the inflamed tissues until you can get proper treatment. KY Jelly is a must. Sexual activity on holiday is usually a top priority! Aci-jel will help to prevent thrush. When it is used at the first signs of an impending attack it may destroy the fungus before it properly takes a hold in the vagina.

If it is possible, ask your doctor if he or she will prescribe a course of anti-fungal pessaries that you can take on holiday. They may not be necessary but it's better to be safe than sorry. Take some minipads in case you have to use the pessaries. If you plan to spend most of your holiday in a bikini, tampons are more discreet. Insert the pessaries at night. Don't use anything to stop the pessary leakage while you are in bed. Allow the melting liquids to do their job. Then use tampons to prevent further leakage during your usual daytime activities. Should you spot the warning signals of a fungal infection while you are away, try to treat it yourself with your emergency provisions. Never wait to see what happens. Mild thrush left untreated will soon develop into acute thrush. Don't swim or bathe. Follow-up a course of pessaries with any sort of self-help remedies that you can acquire, i.e. yoghurt or vinegar-soaked tampons. These will also help to prevent recurrent attacks.

The checklist is only a basic guide. The amount of emergency supplies you need to take with you really depends on the length of time you will be away. If you are going for more than a month, and you anticipate thrush, take lots of pessaries with you, or at least as many as your doctor will prescribe.

If you prepare for the worst, there is no reason why an attack of thrush should ruin your holiday. Relax and enjoy yourself. If you have the opportunity, sun the vulva. It may do the power of good. But be careful not to burn yourself!

A Way of Life

Lifestyle

Looking after your body and your health plays an important role in self-help with thrush. Our hectic lifestyles are very often detrimental to our well-being. Thrush is sometimes referred to as a 'nervous disease', which probably explains why some thrush sufferers are cruelly and mistakenly labelled as 'neurotic'. When we are feeling run down, or under considerable pressure, we have less resistance to invading organisms. Anxiety is a primary cause of psychological stress, and can be a cause of thrush.

Over-exertion drains us. Insufficient sleep, junk food and too much alcohol weaken our defences against infection. When we burn the candle at both ends the body quickly begins to object. Keeping fit and staying healthy will improve the body's ability to fight disease. And exercise will increase the amount of stress that we are able to tolerate. Channelling nervous energy into any form of exercise provides an excellent outlet for anxiety and tension. Exercise will help both your body and your mind to relax. And exercise can be fun too!

Getting rid of thrush can be very difficult. It may take time and it will certainly require a lot of effort. Like other fungal infections, thrush tends to recur. Treating the *symptoms* of thrush won't protect you against further attacks. The *causes* of the infection must be treated too. Generally speaking, anyone who 'suffers' from thrush will always be prone to disease. With a better understanding of your body, by learning to recognise the causes of your particular thrush problem and learning to avoid them, thrush can be overcome. Even though there may be occasional bout of thrush, your new awareness will help you to judge what you can treat yourself and what may need some medical help. In your battle against thrush, preventative care must become a way of life. So keep at it – it will be worth it in the end!

Checklist

There are many reasons why we get thrush. This checklist can be used as a quick reference guide to help you identify the cause(s) of your particular thrush problem. The notes in the right-hand column suggest ways of avoiding further attacks – where they relate to a specific cause:

Possible Causes

YOUR HEALTH
Recent illness?
Antibiotics? Run down?
Not enough sleep?
Other vaginal infections?
Flagyl?

Pregnant?
Diabetes?

Menopause?
Cervical erosion/eversion?

CONTRACEPTION
The Pill

IUD trouble?
Spermicides? Allergy?

SEX
Infection/reinfection from
sexual partner?

Prevention

Avoid antibiotics where-ever this is possible. If you have to take tablets, ask your doctor for a course of thrush pessaries to take concurrently with them.

Ask for a full glucose tolerance test.

Ask for referral to a gynaecologist.

Change brands. Try the progestogen-only pill. A short break from the pill might help.
Visit a family planning clinic for advice on alternative contraception.

Always make sure that your sexual partner or partners are treated when you have thrush. Using a sheath may prevent reinfection.

Alkaline Semen	Sheath. Aci-jel
Prolonged/vigorous inter-course?	KY Jelly

DIET

Poor eating habits?	Read Chapter 7 again.
Junk food?	Yoghurt and vitamin B
Too many sweets/	rich foods will help
sugary foods?	increase vitamin B intake.
Cheese? Mushrooms?	Try rotating diet to isolate
Alcohol?	'suspect' foods. Avoid
	these foods in future.

MISCELLANEOUS

Tights? Nylon pants?	Stockings/suspender (crotchless) tights, cotton pants.
Tight jeans?	Wear skirts instead of trousers.
Exercise in sportswear made of synthetic fibres?	Wear loose-fitting cotton clothes (shorts, skirts etc.)
Nylon leotard?	
Swimming?	Shower after swimming.
Long baths?	Take showers instead of baths.
Vaginal deodorants?	Read Chapters 3 and 11
Deodorised tampons/ towels?	again.
Antiseptics in bath water?	
Bubble baths?	
Over-washing?	
Reinfection from wash cloths?	
Reinfection from bowel?	

On a Final Note . . .

In 1981, the number of people suffering from thrush rose by six per cent. The incidence of thrush is increasing, and it will continue to do so while doctors prescribe antibiotic tablets of ever-increasing strengths, while the pill is promoted as the 'only' contraceptive, while women, persuaded by women's magazines, continue to buy vaginal deodorants and deodorised sanitary protection, and as long as tights and tight jeans remain in fashion. As a result of all this, and in an effort to curb thrush, the drug companies are producing high-powered pessaries and anti-fungal potions, with promises of a faster and more effective relief. The scope of these drugs is limited. Sadly, the relief that they provide is often only temporary. Although the shorter courses of modern treatments can, and do, get rid of thrush very quickly, they cannot and will not solve the problem of recurrent thrush.

It seems unlikely that scientists will ever produce the ultimate cure for thrush. By following the advice set out in this book it is possible to achieve that cure for yourself. Self-help can control thrush and self-help will prevent re-infection. Even during pregnancy, when vaginal thrush can be so hard to shift, self-help will relieve attacks and reduce them to a minimum.

Because thrush often fails to respond to conventional medicine alone, self-help is vital. Much of what you will have read here ought to be common knowledge. If we were given more information on this subject, thrush would cease to be such a distressing and miserable complaint. In the past, women have had to find out about thrush the hard way. Now the simple solution is within easy reach.

Further Reading

The New Women's Health Handbook, edited by Nancy MacKeith, Virago, 1978.

Our Bodies, Ourselves, Angela Phillips and Jill Rakusen, Penguin 1981.

Vaginal Health, Carol Horos, Tobey Dell, 1975.

From Woman to Woman, Lusienne Lanson, Pelican Books, 1977.

Cystitis – The Complete Self-Help Guide, Angela Kilmartin, Hamlyn, 1980.

Understanding Cystitis, Angela Kilmartin, Heinemann, 1973.

Herpes: What to do When You Have It, Dr Oscar Gillespie, Sheldon Press, 1983.

Herbs For Feminine Ailments, Sarah Beckett, Thorsons, 1973.

Let's Get Well, Adelle Davis, Unwin Paperbacks, 1977.

Index